Sickness Work

Gerhard Nijhof

Sickness Work

Personal Reflections of a Sociologist

palgrave
macmillan

Gerhard Nijhof
University of Amsterdam
Amsterdam, The Netherlands

Translated by Nancy Forest-Flier

ISBN 978-981-13-0325-8 ISBN 978-981-13-0326-5 (eBook)
https://doi.org/10.1007/978-981-13-0326-5

Library of Congress Control Number: 2018939733

Printed on acid-free paper

This Palgrave Pivot imprint is published by the registered company Springer Nature Singapore Pte Ltd. part of Springer Nature
The registered company address is: 152 Beach Road, #21-01/04 Gateway East, Singapore 189721, Singapore

For Marga, Piotr, and Eva

Foreword

At the end of 1995, Gerhard Nijhof, medical sociologist, was diagnosed with intestinal cancer in an advanced stage. It meant a turning point in his personal *and* academic life. In early 1996, he was hospitalized for one month, undergoing several difficult operations. He then spent the next twelve months recovering and recuperating at home. During that year, he tried to decipher the notes he had scribbled down while in the hospital, which resulted in the publication in 2001 of a sociologically substantiated autobiographical account of his experiences in the hospital and at home, and what it means to be a seriously ill person. The writing, he remembers, was an integral part of his rehabilitation. This book is a translation and slightly revised version of the Dutch original.

Nijhof first studied medicine, but after one year he turned to sociology. His doctoral dissertation dealt with the relationship between social class and mental disturbances in the city of Rotterdam, which was followed by several books and many articles on this topic. More recently he focused his attention on language and text in the field of health and health care, in particular doctor–patient communication and the life stories of people with chronic diseases. From 1980 to 2003, he was a professor of Medical Sociology at the University of Amsterdam. In 2003, he retired from the university but continued writing and publishing.

Nijhof wrote this autobiographical account of his life as a patient for a wide audience and in deceptively simple language, "deceptively" because his reflection is also addressed to sociologists and other social scientists. It deals with the crucial epistemological question: Is it possible to understand and describe the experiences of those we study, in particular the suffering of the seriously ill? Scientists may make all kinds of claims about what sick people think and feel, but sometimes the sick know from their own experience that they are wrong; the researcher was perhaps fooled by his informants, or he misunderstood them because he did not have any affinity with their experience. Patients and other "experience experts" increasingly criticize researchers for not speaking their language, not picking up the issues that concern them, and not providing information and recommendations that are important to them. Instead, researchers are mostly writing for an academic audience and appear to be much less involved with and close to the people they study than they claim in their prefaces and conclusions. Participation in the anthropological sense of the term would be a more solid and true-to-life basis for the sociological study of sickness and suffering. But is it possible to participate in being a patient?

There are mainly three options for attempting to participate: As patient, as caregiver, or as concerned third party (relative, friend, and visitor), which implies three different roles. The last two are relatively easy; the first—the most relevant one—is, however, extremely difficult and tricky. For experiencing the experiences of the sick person, one cannot content oneself with walking between the beds like a doctor, nurse, or visitor; such a researcher should be a bedridden patient himself. In an earlier publication, Nijhof wrote: "Who knows best what is going on in the minds of dying people? The person who practices participant observation with compassion? Or the one who is close to the sick person? Or the interviewer who inquires into his recent experiences? Or the person who falls sick himself, who thinks about his condition and writes down what happens?" These are rhetorical questions; everyone agrees that the sick person is the best "equipped" "researcher" (provided, of course, that the patient is able to write reflectively about his experiences). Examples of sick people as researchers are, however, relatively scarce.

Two well-known examples of such researchers who were affected by a serious sickness and used their experience to write more empathically and more intelligently about illness are Arthur Frank and Robert Murphy. Murphy (1987) wrote about his illness over a period of eighteen years, from the moment the first symptoms of a spinal cord tumor presented themselves to his being restricted to a wheelchair and becoming entirely dependent on others. This ethnography about one person shows what illness does to social identity. His struggle for autonomy slowly grows into acceptance and finding deeper meaning. His reflection starts with an observation from the time when he still was an outsider to the world of disease and disability. He sees a severely disabled person in a wheelchair and wonders why such a person would want to live. He is unable to grasp that person's desire for life. When, many years later, he is disabled himself, he remembers that moment and is finally able to explain to himself and his readers how much life still holds for him.

Arthur Frank (1991, 2001, 2004) has written extensively about his own experiences of illness, using them as "data" that enhance his authority as an author of sickness and suffering. He (Frank 2001) takes the position of a patient who is approached by a researcher; that meeting can lead to feelings of disrespect and insult if the sick person feels he/she is being broken down into ethnographically and theoretically interesting fragments.

Gerhard Nijhof's *Sickness Work* deserves a place in the company of authors such as Frank and Murphy (and several others mentioned in his account). Moreover, it is an attempt from an insider's perspective to forge a new kind of medical sociology. For most medical sociologists, serious illness is not a personal experience. They conduct surveys or hold interviews and return to their universities or homes to analyze and write up their findings. The concepts they use reveal their provenance: the minds of healthy sociologists. Nijhof became acutely aware of this when he fell sick, encountering completely different concepts. One such concept was "techno-security." Social scientists had written extensively and critically about the "technologization" of medical care. Doctors and nurses are criticized for being busier with machines than with people. The machine becomes the patient's enemy, or at least his/her rival. Nijhof had rarely read anything about the sense of security that machines may bring to patients. For him, alternatively, the machines were sources of trust and security, magical instruments that kept him alive. When, shortly after his operation, a doctor told him the "good news" that he could leave the intensive care unit and return to the ward, he was scared. He did not want to be separated from the safety that the machines provided.

Another new focus point was the night as an unresearched or undiscussed phenomenon, unacknowledged in medical sociology, which only seemed to be interested in daylight. "I cannot remember ever having come across the word 'night' in any of my literature. Most sociologists sleep at night, and society is closed for them then. But perhaps night is absent from their work because they think little happens there, they think other people sleep at night, too. But that is a mistake." One of the disruptions of everyday life brought about by sickness is that the rhythm of day and night is interrupted. "It's no longer a matter of working during the day and sleeping at night. You don't work anymore. You sleep whenever sleep overtakes you, if you can fall asleep, and not if you can't fall asleep." Getting through the night is one of the most difficult tasks of "sickness work." The television, with its repetitions of daytime programs such as political discussions, football matches, tennis tournaments, and the Tour de France, saved him. His reflections on the night end in a plea for "every-night healthcare" (in contrast to "every-day").

A recurrent theme in his musings as well as in his most recent work, including his valedictory lecture (Nijhof 2004), are the concepts of normality and everydayness. "Sickness work" is a matter of changing the abnormality of being disabled and fragile into normality. "This book is mainly about technique, about the work of learning to do unusual things in an ordinary way, about developing routines," he writes. And: "Everything that had seemed exciting and unusual at first turned out to be quite ordinary after a brief stay." Recapturing normality, one could say, is a way of regaining a new form of "health." Abnormality is perhaps the most outspoken telltale sign of sickness. This thought is the central intuition of his later work on Parkinson's disease (e.g., Nijhof 1995).

His main "conversion" as a sociologist was his acknowledgment of the importance of the unspoken word. For years he had been studying words, spoken and written. Analyzing texts had been his main occupation, until he came to realize that people may keep silent about certain experiences. "When sociologists conduct interviews, they usually focus on the talk and rarely on the silence. We know that people are silent about a great many things, but it's their talking that we listen to. It's true that we encourage them to talk, but the things that people keep their mouths shut about escape us." That is the reason that interrogating sociologists miss so much of what sickness means to sick people. A sickness such as cancer is mainly surrounded by silence...

It should be noted that Nijhof wrote his reflections mostly in 1996 and that they were published in 2001. His critical comments about the status of his own discipline, medical sociology, must be placed within that period. Most of the shortcomings he called attention to, such as ignoring the night, the problem of fatigue, the work of nurses, the verticality of the horizontal patient, the trust in technology, the silence of suffering—in short, the patient's point of view—have since received considerable attention from medical sociologists and anthropologists. One could therefore say that his suggestions for a more true-to-life sociology were prophetic. The absence of present-day sociologists in his references should be seen in that light. No update has been attempted in this English translation of his work. The book takes us back to the year 1996 but also makes us wonder about today.

The main merit of Nijhof's book lies in the personal and professional reflection on one case of sickness, and taking that one case as a vantage point from which to explore wider areas in the experience of being critically ill. His story is similar to autobiographical accounts of colleagues such as Irving Zola, Robert Murphy, Arthur Frank, and Albert Robillard. Each of these authors had a specific focus; Nijhof's central experience and idea—as I just mentioned—was that the rupture of normality and everyday routine brought about by sickness had to be reversed through hard work and continuous readjustment. His account of the small details and imponderabilia of everyday navigation within the restrictions of sickness is as relevant today as it was in 1996.

Nijhof's pondering shows what the radical sharing of experience brings about in research on the meaning of sickness. Participating in sickness cannot be programmed, but when one falls sick, one may make a "virtue" out of this necessity. *Permanent receptivity* by the patient is the most felicitous way to achieve intersubjectivity in research, but sickness is at the same time a personal misfortune, a condition that obstructs research. Permanent receptivity of one's own condition helps one to grasp the opportunity to come closer to "the other." Frank (2004: 439) captures this permanent receptivity by turning around the well-known counsel that the researcher should go where the action is. We should rather be aware that there is "action" wherever we are, he argues. Gerhard Nijhof's reflection is an impressive example of this receptivity while being seriously sick. In the eminent translation by Nancy Forest-Flier, this book is both a testimony to sharing the intimate experience of sickness with others and a humble prolegomenon of a more experience-based medical sociology.

Amsterdam, The Netherlands

Sjaak van der Geest
Emeritus Professor of
Medical Anthropology

References

Frank, A. 1991. *At the Will of the Body: Reflections on Illness*. Boston: Houghton Mifflin.

Frank, A. 2001. Can We Research Suffering? *Qualitative Health Research* 11 (3): 353–362.

Frank, A. 2004. After Methods, the Story: From Incongruity to Truth in Qualitative Research. *Qualitative Health Research* 14 (3): 430–440.

Murphy, R. 1987. *The Body Silent*. New York: Norton.

Nijhof, G. 1995. Parkinson's Disease as a Problem of Shame in Public Appearance. *Sociology of Health & Illness* 17 (2): 193–205.

Nijhof, G. 2004. *Ongewoon Ziekenleven. Afscheidscollege* [Unusual Sick Life. Valedictory Lecture]. Amsterdam: Het Spinhuis.

Preface

I spent thirty years working as a medical sociologist, but I had never been ill before. Suddenly that changed. I was diagnosed with cancer. Almost immediately my illness became an object of research. That's the beauty of sociology: You can do it anywhere and anytime. Even during the first nights after my operation, I was giving sociology lectures in my morphine dreams. Those morphine-induced lectures grew into a whole series, and at a certain point I guessed I had forty lectures all told. But how to remember them all? Write them down, I said to myself. But in the middle of the night, when you're all doped up, how do you lay your hands on a pen and paper? I knew there were some writing supplies in one of my drawers. After rummaging around, I found what I was looking for and wrote down whatever it was I thought was so important.

Several days later, after a great deal of decoding, I figured out what I had written: "gift nurse" and "they treat us here like lunatics." There was more, but it was illegible. The first message was easy. It had to do with an intensive care nurse who, with great solicitude, had succeeded in bringing me back to the land of the living. Why is so much attention paid to doctors in medical sociology and so little to nurses, I wondered, now that my head was clear. A lecture! The second message took much longer to unravel. That had to do with my stay in the recovery room when I was still half under following the first operation and awaiting the second, and I dreamt that right next to my bed a male nurse was doing repairs on his motorbike and leaving me and a groaning woman next to me completely unattended. No lecture on that subject. Teaching requires a sober mind!

Yet it kept eating at me. What were those other thirty-eight lectures about? One year later I took another sober look at what had happened to me. I wasn't going to make it to forty, although I did get up to twenty-four. I had written them over a period of two weeks, when I was down with a nasty cold. Little ailments like that hit me much harder than they had before my illness. I got up and took two aspirin for my headache and fever, which gave me an hour and a half of discomfort-free writing time. I sat down at my PC without a topic or purpose in mind. I thought for a second. Then I typed whatever came into my head. There was always a story attached. The first story I typed sank into oblivion due to a computer crash. It was, I thought, the most important thing I had to say, but I've never been able to remember anything about it. A total write-off. The rest of the stories survived, however. They have become this book.

Once they were typed out, my experiences turned into stories. The act of typing was a way of processing what had happened to me, a kind of psychotherapy. Only afterward did I attempt to see the stories sociologically, and then they became research data. For the past twenty-five years, I have been examining the impact of chronic illness on people's lives with the aid of their life stories. Now, through my own life stories, I am examining that impact up close. As I continued, I added introductions and drew conclusions. Thus the stories became more than what psychologists call "processing." For a sociologist like me, they became signs of that special competence that is unique to humans: taking the unfamiliar for granted. Being ill is like traveling: After one week, Morocco becomes quite routine.

I am not the only one who has told stories about his illness. Many have done it before me. At first such stories were told by other people, usually people who were closely involved with the sick person. But more recently it has been the sick themselves who have taken up the pen. One publisher estimated that a quarter of the manuscripts sent to him had to do with the life stories of sick people. Those who collect such stories, as I do professionally, soon have a shelf full of them. What follows is a modest selection. John Hull writes about his life with blindness in his *Touching the Rock*, Robert McCrum talks about his life after a stroke in *My Year Off*. In Andy Murcia and Bob Stewart's *Man to Man: When the Woman you Love has Breast Cancer*, two married couples tell their stories. And Patricia Duncker and Vicky Wilson's *Cancer* contains the stories of ten individual women.

Sociologists—and anthropologists, too—have preceded me in writing about their lives with illness. In 1982, the American Irving Zola wrote about his experiences as a disabled person living in "Het Dorp," a village for the disabled in the Netherlands, in his *Missing Pieces: A Chronicle of Living with a Disability*. The first sociological analysis of an author's own illness that I know of is by the American sociologist Lefton, who in 1984 explored his experiences with Parkinson's disease in *Chronic Disease and Applied Sociology: An Essay in Personalized Sociology*. This was followed in 1987 by the anthropologist Robert Murphy, whose *The Body Silent* contains an analysis of his reaction, and that of others, to his paraplegia resulting from a tumor on his spinal cord. In 1991, Arthur Frank subjected his experiences with cancer and a heart attack to sociological investigation in *At the Will of the Body*. In 1993, Sally French analyzed her life with blindness in *Can You See the Rainbow?* And in 1999, the ethnomethodologist Albert Robillard published an autobiographical analysis of his life with ALS in *Meaning of Disability*. Obviously, social scientists do not stop being what they are when they become ill.

All this writing about illness is not so very remarkable. Illness upsets one's ordinary routine; illness attacks our innocence. Illness violates the hard core of society: Our unquestioned acceptance that things will keep going as they always have gone. Illness interrupts us in our "natural attitude" (Schutz 1962). Such a violation generates unease, as well as introspection. But illness does more than that to people. Illness also means setting foot in unknown territory, with all the travel experiences that go with it.

But why do all these sick people write about their illnesses? Apparently there is little shame involved in personal suffering. But perhaps another reason sick people write is because they realize that illness often brings something else with it: The unexpected capacity to overcome difficulties, for example. Life stories of the sick are not always heart-warming, however. They also contain complaints about what has been done to them: The recklessness of those who caused the condition, the inattentiveness of doctors, and the incomprehension of outsiders. Often there's also a desire to reveal what's going on behind the scenes: Unusual experiences, the fight for a decent life, and the difficulties with which many sick people are saddled. This transforms individual suffering into a social question.

Sick people are often banished from the public eye. They find themselves in the back rooms of society. By telling their life stories, they publicize what otherwise would remain private. But their stories do more than that. To write an autobiography is to legitimize one's experience. When sick people tell their life stories they are both explaining and justifying them, they are making them transparent. With their stories, they are challenging what many sociologists have observed among the long-term sick: incomprehension.

I am also trying to do medical sociology with my stories, and for several reasons. The first is personal. As a sick person you're sometimes bewildered by your own behavior—and that of others. I use medical-sociological concepts to make my own confusing experiences more intelligible.

There is also a second personal reason. When I write about my experiences, I feel somewhat exposed. I don't talk about my illness without a certain apprehension. I try to hide that apprehension behind my sociological comments. My discipline is good for many things, but hiding the personal sometimes goes a bit too far. So I write about being ill in general, even though I'm only talking about *my* life with *my* illness. That kind of generalization simply will not do. Read it as a proposal for further research.

The third reason is my suspicion that analyzing the personal experiences of the sick can also contribute to the development of medical sociology. Serious illness is something that most medical sociologists have never experienced firsthand. They study illness from a certain distance, and even more so when they arrange to have sick people interviewed by means of questionnaires. This is characteristic of medical sociology as a whole. Many of the concepts used in medical sociology could only have originated in the heads of healthy sociologists. Few of them are rooted in direct experience with sick people or healthcare professionals. For this reason, I believe that medical sociology can actually benefit from having these experiences put into words. So I am trying to do medical sociology based on my own experience of illness. I describe experiences that medical sociology tends to pass over, and I try to coin new words for such experiences. The result is a personal medical sociology. By examining my own everyday experiences through a sociological lens, I am trying to develop a sociological definition of illness. In my experience, illness is mainly a "disruption of the unquestioned regularity of life." It attacks the everyday innocence that people live with. Sociologically speaking, illness is a "disease of human innocence."

I am also using this sociological commentary on my experience of illness to try to interest readers in medical sociology. For those whose interest is piqued, I have included notes with references. I have been somewhat personal in my choice of literature and refer quite frequently to my own work. That is because this slim volume brings together the things that interest me: the medical sociology of the chronically ill and the method of life story research.

Finally, I have linked my experiences to the way the healthcare system is organized. I pay particular attention to experiences that the healthcare system does not deal with very well. Illness involves a great deal of mundane work that professional health care is not set up to handle. As a result, sick people have to do a lot of that work themselves: "sickness work."

By definition, medical sociology has to do with the phenomena of people thinking and speaking in terms of "illness," "health," and "health care," things to which they attach medical meanings and often deal with medically. That attribution of medical meanings is not limited to people in health care alone. Ordinary people do the same thing in their day-to-day lives. But very often they attribute other meanings as well, interpreting in terms of their own feelings and sometimes on their own authority. The meanings that sick people themselves attach to what is happening to them are often relegated to second place. Doctors do this fairly often. They have every right to do so because it's their profession, a profession that we have conferred on them—by legal means, in fact. But that doesn't prevent ordinary people from interpreting things in their own way. These interpretations are sometimes of lesser importance to doctors, but that isn't true for ordinary people—sick people, for example. People use their own interpretations to construct their social reality, and they live within the reality of these interpretations. Such interpretations form the social reality that is the basis of their lives. The interpretations that people ascribe to the phenomena of body and mind are what they live from. They constitute their social reality. That social reality is what sociology is interested in.

This is why I have turned my attention here to the interpretations that I as an ordinary individual ascribe to what happened to me in my experience with intestinal cancer, to the treatment I received, and to the repercussions of that treatment.

It is my hope that by closely watching and listening to myself, the people who live with me, and the professionals who care for me, I can have a positive impact on my life with my illness as well as on my field of medical sociology. This book is too impressionistic to be called science, but it may seem to approach science at times. That is mainly because a sick sociologist sees and hears more than a healthy one does.

Amsterdam, The Netherlands Gerhard Nijhof

Reference

Schutz, A. 1962. *Collected Papers I: The Problem of Social Reality*. The Hague: Nijhoff.

Contents

1 Introduction	1
2 Disruption	9
3 Incantation	21
4 Collective Disruption	33
5 Sickness Work	43
6 Control	67
7 The Outside World	81
8 Legitimation	101
9 Epilogue	113
Bibliography	117
Index	121

CHAPTER 1

Introduction

Abstract This long essay is about what cancer did to my everyday existence, and especially about how I, and the people who live with me, responded to my illness. It is also an account of how personal experiences changed my vision of medical sociology. The aim of this essay can be seen in its design. In twenty-three vignettes or subchapters, I describe typical experiences of being sick and try to (re)locate them within the sociological discourse.

Keywords Reflection · Illness experience · Medical sociology

This little book is all about being ill, but not in the medical sense of the word. I don't describe my illness the way doctors do. It's also not about what the doctors and nurses did to me; it's not about operations and treatments. It's about what illness did to my everyday existence, and especially about what I, and the people who live with me, did with me and my illness. What that essentially meant was "work": ordinary work.[1] "Sickness work" made my illness an ordinary illness.

Using the term "work" to apply to what sick people do when they are ill is taken from the publications of Anselm Strauss and his fellow researchers. They, of all medical sociologists, have been the most persistent in focusing attention on the complex and comprehensive work that such sick people undertake in order to make their illness livable.

G. Nijhof, *Sickness Work*,
https://doi.org/10.1007/978-981-13-0326-5_1

Their basic premise was the assertion that illness is not just "experienced." More importantly, it is something to be "managed."

As a medical sociologist, I knew the social dimensions of getting ill and being ill, as well as the treatment of illness. But as it turned out there was a great deal I did not know. I soon discovered that medical sociology is just as dominated by the medical world as care of the sick is. The doctors and nurses appeared to know a great deal about illness and medicine, but they knew much less about "everyday illness" and the "everyday" aspects of living with illness, and medical sociologists don't know much more. The medical bias of both these groups causes them to suffer from what Robert Merton calls "trained incapacity," an acquired inability to see what sick people are up against every day.

After being in the hospital for less than a day I saw how much medical sociologists tend to overlook. Medical sociology is mainly about doctors, while most of my contacts were with nurses. Medical sociology is mainly about interactions between doctors and patients, but when I was in the hospital what I heard and saw was that my doctors didn't talk to me as much as they talked with others about me. Sometimes that happened right outside my door, in conversations with nurses and ward physicians. I heard things they didn't tell me later on, and if they did tell me, it was often something slightly different. Sometimes I heard that they had talked with fellow specialists, but inpatient consultations, which are even further removed. I heard nothing about these meetings, or a brief summary at the most. Sometimes I saw two or three standing nearby and mumbling to each other, sometimes behind glass walls. Sometimes one of them might notify me of findings or plans. Sometimes I heard casual discussions casually taking place between doctors. But most of all I saw knowing glances, those interactions that sociologists cannot capture with their tape recorders. And medical sociologists seem to know nothing at all about nurses: The nurses who look over at you during a consultation and later say, "That was typical Doctor A," or "That seems a little too soon to me; let's wait and do it tomorrow." I can only guess what their reasons are, reasons they don't usually express in the presence of doctors. But later on I saw and heard what they did. And then there are the interactions with countless other hospital staff: Research doctors, nameless laboratory technicians, dieticians, the laboratory researchers who take and study blood samples, roommates and their visitors.

I also saw what it is that influences treatment: The essentials and the side issues, the specialisms and whatever falls outside it, the focus on success and the avoidance of failure, the chance of prestige if the treatment is successful, and the difference between the disease and related incidents, such as infections.

Only a little of what I heard and saw was recognizable from my work as a medical sociologist. I noticed that some doctors did things one way and some of them another, that there were doctors who talked and doctors who were silent, that some appealed to experience and intuition and others to test results, that some had more authority than others, that some nurses took me in hand and others kept their distance, that some of them were more focused on the machines and others on my body and others on me, and some on all three, one after another, or even all three at the same time. I saw some of them much more than others, and a few I never saw again. And mainly I saw how much information ended up on my hospital chart without anyone having asked me any questions.

What I saw was everyday health care. And what I and the people around me later did was everyday health care. I saw myself monkeying around with things that I had never been interested in before: The machines and tubes attached to my body. And I qualified what many of the people around me were doing to me as "sickness work." I saw sickness work as mainly the occupation of my wife Mar and myself. She organized and I tinkered, as if that was our ultimate passion. We had no choice. There was no avoiding it.

When sociologists study the care of the sick, they're mainly thinking about others. That fits right in with the healthcare culture in which we live. Care is something that somebody else does. We may hear more and more about "self-care," but that takes place outside the healthcare realm. Only recently has self-care been brought to public attention, mainly through the writings of the sick themselves.

But sickness work is not practiced by the sick alone. When sickness struck, my wife and I had to figure out what was going on. What kind of illness was it? How far advanced? How virulent? And: who is a good surgeon? And later: where is the illness going to take us?

And even later, in the hospital: what are our chances? Who knows what? But also: how do I get through the night? What medicines help? What do I respond to badly? What shots would be catastrophic for me? And how can I get them discontinued? What pills put me to sleep? What should I tell the doctors? And what do I keep to myself? How do we find out what we want to know? Whom should we tackle with our questions: The ward physician, a nurse, my surgeon, or none of the above?

One of their colleagues perhaps? How are you to interpret their faces? What are they really saying if they refuse to talk about something? Can you ask the nurses what you haven't asked the doctors? How do you lie in bed without pain? But equally important were the questions about our—new—everyday life. What do we need to learn in order to live with the illness? How do we get through the day, and the night? How do we become accustomed to the effects of the illness? How do we conceal the vestiges of the surgical procedures? How do we learn to live with the impediments that the illness saddles us with? All these were things that Mar and I had to figure out. We learned to manage the situation as circumstances required.

This didn't change when I was released from the hospital. In fact it only intensified. Mar and I had to learn how to deal with the illness and come to an understanding, not only with the illness but also with each other, Mar with me and I with her, us with my children and they with us, us with my family, with people at work, and with anyone who showed an interest. That's what this book is about: This ordinary, everyday sickness work.

Sickness work is not the work of professionals. The sick people collective is on its own, and its members have to figure things out for themselves. They have to because there is very little official care for everyday sickness. There are homecare programs, but most of them are only available when there's something officially wrong with your body, something that has a name, preferably a medical name. Those who advocate home care—mostly as a way of saving money—also talk about "voluntary home care" when appropriate, by which they usually mean the partner and the children. The main problem for the architects of a voluntary homecare policy is that more and more people don't have partners to turn to. And even if they do, the homecare advocates don't seem to realize that often the partner simply cannot be there—because he or she works, for example, or because they have their own commitments, their own lives to manage.

Often the sick person and his or her partner—if they have one—are alone in the day-to-day necessity of grappling with the illness that has confronted them. And after a while they know better than anyone else what their problems are and how to cope with them. In addition, these problems often occur at times when official healthcare workers are unavailable (read: asleep), or they occur in places where healthcare workers don't go, such as bathrooms or bedrooms. Simply by doing this everyday sickness work, the sick person and his partner become more adept than official healthcare workers ever could be.

The paradox of being ill is that sick people become dependent on others and at the same time are thrown back on themselves. I could not have managed without the help of other people. If I had been alone, I never would have come through my illness alive. But without myself I couldn't have managed either.

Sickness seems to bring out the best in people. Right from the first day, an army of doctors and nurses snapped to attention, detailed examinations were performed on me and incisions were expertly made, IV drips were put in place on my body, sandwiches were made for me, and my pillows were fluffed. But an army of homecare personnel was also working nonstop: Friends were informed, a bed was brought in, I was cheered up, I was fed, Mar organized her life around mine. That was all the work of other people.

I did very little, especially in the beginning. What I mainly tried to do was not to become a burden to everyone else, but even that was more than I could manage at first. Eventually, however, I began to knuckle down. After only three days I started washing myself, and from then on I did more and more on my own. I tinkered with my body—mostly with the things that were attached to it—as if I were managing a small refinery. I organized my medications. I tried to get my bowel movements under control. I tried to see how far I could walk. I talked about my illness, explaining to people what I had done, and especially what I hadn't done. I tried to get through each ordinary day doing ordinary sickness work.

That's what this book is about: Doing that work, the work I did alone, that others did with me and I with them. It isn't work of the highest order for the most part. What the body mainly requires is maintenance, doing what it needs at that particular moment. The sick person and his partner, if there is one and if he or she is available, will be spending quite some time on the staff of the maintenance and cleaning service of the State of the Sick. Most of this involves learning: Learning all over again how to keep house and how to live together in a way that is acceptable to you both, and relearning what you hadn't given much thought to since childhood: Walking, strolling, climbing stairs, sleeping in an ordinary bed, and knowing what makes you tired. But then it gets even more difficult: Coming to an understanding with the people who are involved in your life. That calls for a great deal of attention, as well as a lot of explaining and justifying, a lot of "legitimation."[2] That is the work that the sick person has to learn, as does anyone who may be close to him.

This book is mainly about myself. Any others mentioned here are seen through my eyes: The eyes of a sick person, a sick person who was not used to having much to do with other people. So being ill was a two-pronged confrontation for me: I saw myself tinkering not only with myself but also with others. That tinkering taught me a lot: about myself and about sociology. And it was through all that tinkering that this book emerged as a medical sociological case study. Such a case study turns sociology into a personal undertaking. Although it runs the risk of being overly personal, the benefit of this endeavor is that you become thoroughly familiar with the research data. Many sociological researchers distance themselves from whatever it is they're researching, mainly by using standardized questionnaires and remote statistical data processing procedures. But even sociologists who engage in the method of "participatory observation" often go no further than participating in the lives of others. Personal sociology has its limitations, of course. Not every sociologist can become the subject of his own study. But illness touches the lives of most sociologists sooner or later, which is why there have already been several firsthand sociological studies of illness, as I mentioned before (Lefton 1984; Murphy 1987; Frank 1991; Robillard 1999).

The aim of this book can be seen in its design. Each chapter contains several "subchapters" and each subchapter describes a typical experience in three steps. I begin by searching for hints in the medical sociological literature in order to help me locate that experience. Then I describe the experience itself. My interpretation of the experience was the social reality of my illness. The third step is my search for a way to characterize the experience in sociological terms, and my attempt to find a word for it. Usually that word becomes the title of the subchapter.

In this way, I shaped a personal sociology of my experience of illness. But at the same time, that sociology shaped my life in terms of what happened to me. "There is no other social reality than that which is constructed in the interpretations of those involved," I used to say in my lectures. Now I was experiencing that at firsthand. "Interpretations are not merely personal. They are also guided by the culture in which people live. This provides us with the social grammar by which we articulate what we experience," I would add. My sociology, I discovered, was part of my grammar. Sociologists don't stop being sociologists when they become ill. In my case, I saw how "my" sociology came to shape my life with my illness.

Notes

1. The "everydayness" of sickness work is pointed out by Corbin and Strauss (1988) in their notions of the work of managing illness: "sickness work," "everyday work," "biographical work," and "arrangement work."
2. This "legitimation work" of the chronically ill has become one of the main themes of my research after my illness (see Nijhof 1995, 1996, 1998, 2004).

References

Corbin, J., and A. Strauss. 1988. *Unending Work and Care: Managing Chronic Illness at Home*. San Francisco and London: Jossey-Bass.

Frank, A. 1991. *At the Will of the Body: Reflections on Illness*. Boston: Houghton Mifflin.

Lefton, M. 1984. Chronic Disease and Applied Sociology: An Essay in Personalised Sociology. *Sociological Inquiry* 54: 466–476.

Murphy, R. 1987. *The Body Silent*. New York: Norton.

Nijhof, G. 1995. Parkinson's Disease as a Problem of Shame in Public Appearance. *Sociology of Health & Illness* 17 (2): 193–205.

Nijhof, G. 1996. Uncertainty and Lack of Trust with Parkinson's Disease. *European Journal of Public Health* 6 (1): 58–63.

Nijhof, G. 1998. Heterogeneity in the Interpretation of Epilepsy. *Qualitative Health Research* 8 (1): 95–105.

Nijhof, G. 2004. *Ongewoon Ziekenleven. Afscheidscollege* [Unusual Sick Life. Valedictory Lecture]. Amsterdam: Het Spinhuis.

Robillard, A. 1999. *Meaning of Disability: The Lived Experience of Paralysis*. Philadelphia: Temple University Press.

CHAPTER 2

Disruption

Abstract Sickness causes disruption to one's normal existence. In this chapter I discuss three moments of this disruption. The first is the bad news message. That message does not merely consist of words, as sociologists usually assume, but also of unspoken hints and gestures. The second is that bad news interrupts our everyday "naivety"; lots of things cease to be taken for granted and require extra effort from the sick person. The third is that confusion and continuous fatigue take over, conditions that do not really interest medical professionals, which further exacerbates the patient's feeling of being lost.

Keywords Bad news · Innocence · Fatigue

The Bad News Gesture

Bad news is carried by way of conversation, sociologists say.[1] At least that's what I gather from the studies I've read on the subject. This idea is firmly embedded in our linguistic culture. We take it for granted that bad news is expressed in terms of language.

That is why medical sociologists are mainly interested in how "bad news conversations" are conducted (see e.g., Taylor 1988). Doctors tend to formulate their messages with great care, to begin them with an introduction and to end them with a conclusion. But there are also those who like to keep it short, who come right out with the bad news.

G. Nijhof, *Sickness Work*,
https://doi.org/10.1007/978-981-13-0326-5_2

My doctor's style was different than anything I had ever read about, and shorter, too.

* * *

Man does not live by language alone, a fact that was made brutally clear to me. I had been in this hospital before. One year earlier I had a sudden heavy hemorrhage while sitting on the toilet. That's it for me, was my immediate reaction. My mother had greeted me with the same announcement twenty years ago when I called her after returning home from vacation. Six months later she was dead.

I was referred to a surgeon—an assistant surgeon, as I later found out. His boss was away in Japan on a study trip, he told me by way of explanation. He examined my intestines with a scope and diagnosed a ruptured blood vessel in the intestinal wall. "Other hospitals would patch it up," he added. "We just leave it alone." Feeling properly defended, I left the hospital with my mind at ease.

One year later there was another incident of bleeding. It barely fazed me. "Now they *will* have to patch it up," I said to myself, suspecting nothing. Back I went to the hospital. The first person I saw was the assistant from the year before. He saw me, too, and slipped behind a filing cabinet—rather hastily, I thought. The senior surgeon examined me in the same way: on my knees, bent over. He inserted the scope in my rectum. He was standing behind me where I couldn't see him. The examination was over in five minutes. He washed his hands. Walked past me. Gave my arm a squeeze. "This is bad" I thought. His gesture shot through me like an electrical charge. "You can get dressed now." No sooner was I back in my clothes than he walked right up to me. "It's cancer," he said. I covered my face with my hands. "It's probably operable," is what I later thought I heard him say. He must have said more. I only know that I got lost on the way home. The hospital is about 500 meters from my house, but I no longer knew what street I lived on, or what direction my house was in.

My surgeon did it with a single gesture. Most gestures are appropriate to a given situation. In this particular situation they're quite common. You know what they mean. A squeeze of the arm means that one person is trying to buck the other up, or to comfort him. My surgeon made that gesture. But why did he think such assurance was necessary? Without words, this gesture, in this situation, meant "cancer."

* * *

Why do so many medical sociologists miss gestures like this? Because most of the time we only ask questions and listen, but we rarely look. Sociologists like to conduct interviews and record conversations, but we hardly ever pay attention to how things are happening in practice. Like so many people in our culture, sociologists are language-oriented, not gesture-oriented. We maintain a safe distance from what's actually going on, like a bunch of frightened rabbits. We'd rather ask questions later, when it's all over. In a hospital many things just happen, according to routine, without words. As a patient I saw a lot of this. Being in the hospital trained me well in the sociology of the gesture.

Bearing bad news means breaking through the everyday routine. Bad news is the caesura between before and after. It transforms ordinary life into something else. There are times when we eagerly welcome change. We're only too glad to leave the rat race, to take a short break from our normal lives and go on vacation. But sometimes such a break means that life will never be the same. Sickness, accidents, loss, hospitalization, imprisonment, divorce: these are the kinds of breaks that intrude on our existence. In many cases such breaks are simple matters. They just happen. But sometimes they have to be announced, and that is a tough job. No one is good at it. A few people acquire the skill: police officers, clergymen, doctors, process servers, teachers. But for the recipients of bad news there is no such training program. It's always new. They're taken by surprise. For them it's always a crisis.

In a crisis people are left empty-handed.[2] What do you do when life as you know it is no longer relevant? In such a situation people get lost in their own surroundings, because the bad news renders them strangers.

Innocence Interrupted

Our everyday social life is characterized by an unquestioned acceptance of certain things. We see them as we think they actually are. And usually we think they're going to stay that way. So we take it for granted that something like disease exists, that sick people have diseases, and that doctors practice medicine. We also think that life is going to continue as it always has, that tomorrow is going to be just like today. But—"thinking"? Thinking is just what we don't do when we take something for granted. We regard such a thing as "natural." And we don't think about things that are natural.[3] We don't give a moment's thought to the everyday. We live with it without thinking about it, quite innocently.

The same is true of our bodies. As long as we're healthy, we take it for granted that our bodies will work and that we can do anything we want to with them. We don't notice how much we take our bodies for granted until something goes wrong. Then our innocence pays the price, and that only exacerbates the problems imposed by our malfunctioning bodies. Of course we are unprepared when the things we take for granted break down. And when that does happen our innocence is the first to go.

Many sociologists used rather grand language when they talked about illness. They spoke and still speak of "deviation" (Parsons 1952: 436–439; Scheff 1984), of "loss of independence," of "the shrinking of one's social existence" (Lyons et al. 1995). In doing so they turn illness into something grand, something very different from the ordinary. They give illness a special place of its own. Illness is relegated to places reserved for the sick: usually doctors' offices and hospitals.

But sick people are more ordinary than the language of these sociologists suggests, and they are far more likely to be found outside the waiting room and hospital than inside. They spend a lot of time at home. Most of the time you can't distinguish them from ordinary people, at least not from the outside.

Usually what sets sick people apart are the little things. They come across as people who have trouble doing what they used to take for granted and what others in turn regarded as natural. Sociologically speaking, sickness is a disease of innocence.

Sociologists know that sickness impacts a person's social life. Usually it manifests itself in specific areas of life in terms of ordinary incompetence, limited mobility and a shrunken network, isolation, stigmatization, and dependence on others. But my loss of innocence affected almost everything. For me, sickness turned out to be more imperialistic than many medical sociologists seem to think.

It was through that very interruption of innocence that my illness told me something about normal life, my own and everyone else's, about the innocence with which people generally go through life. Healthy people do things the way they're accustomed to doing them. And when something goes wrong, there are automatic explanations for it. When something hurts, we immediately think, "I've pulled a muscle."

* * *

After a while it dawned on me: I was relating to things differently. I began to see many of them in a new light. It wasn't pronounced, like something you're constantly thinking about. It was more like yeast: It permeated everything. I found myself reflecting on many of the things I was doing. How long would I be able to do what I had just done? Should I keep on doing it? Was it even worth the trouble? Would I be able to finish it if I were to start right now? Would life tomorrow be the same as it once had been? Would it ever be the same? Would I ever be able to just work until I was tired? Would life ever go back to normal? These formulations may be a bit over the top. What I experienced was more blurred, an indistinct feeling that many things had become different, and that I couldn't take them for granted anymore. After a while I found a term for it: my "everyday innocence" was gone. I found myself asking unarticulated questions every time I did something routine. A vague uncertainty wormed its way into my life. Only gradually did I come to realize what the illness was doing to me.

When I became ill, I noticed that life was no longer as simple as it had been. I wondered how far I'd be able to bike, or if I couldn't go back to the last few places where I had spent my youth. And when I started planning a new article, I wondered whether it wouldn't be better to choose a more important topic. I really did write about other things: about the future of my field, for example. Suddenly I became concerned about things that I used to shrug off. I also started working faster, as if I couldn't count on another day following this one. Time had always been a precious commodity for me, but now I knew what it felt like to have no time at all. At nine o'clock on Sunday mornings I'd be sitting at my PC, and whereas I used to stop after an hour or two, now I'd try to squeeze in a little extra time.

I also started thinking differently about death. "Think" is too grand a word for what I was doing. It was more an awareness that slipped into my head, the way you suddenly notice that it's getting dark outside. Life felt different. I think I used to believe that dying was a slow process of steady deterioration, a realization that the end was approaching and that the people around you knew it and had slowly started relating to you differently. Now dying was "falling over the edge." All of a sudden it's over, unexpected, no time to say goodbye. Even with death the innocence of life had disappeared.

The loss of innocence doesn't make life any simpler. I find myself pondering many things that I used to just pass over. This is awkward and tiresome. I really would like to do something again without thinking about it. Sometimes I succeed. Things I do seem to happen of their own accord. I notice that sometimes the sense of the habitual is back, that the illness is losing its control.

This feeling is reinforced by going on vacation. After two years I made my first getaway. I didn't know what hit me. I wandered around, feeling completely uninhibited. It was another world, another self. I hadn't realized until then that I was seeing flashes of my sickness-centered life in many of the things inside my house. The house itself evoked them. *That* was the toilet where I saw the first signs of my illness. That was the place where I had spent so much time flat on my back. That was the radio program I listened to kill time. There was the hallway where I tried to walk after my operation. That was my study, the place where I moved the books around at night after my illness was diagnosed. Those daily associations don't stand a chance on vacation. That's where innocence gains ground.

Gradually I was also beginning to understand what my strategy was for keeping this interrupted innocence outside my head: by making sure my head was full, working hard, leaving no time for fantasizing. But even with that realization the world will always be a little different. I don't believe that the everyday innocence from the past will ever return.

* * *

It's strange that as a sociologist I had never noticed that the world consists of routine and innocence until I became ill. That's because I myself am a creature of routine and innocence, of course. I didn't see that until I found myself somewhat removed from society, until I left the domain of the healthy. Sick people are better than healthy ones at seeing the habitual on which society is founded.

Sociology exists by virtue of the routine, however. Without the things we take for granted there would be no society, and hence no sociology. But it's precisely because of that routine that we focus so little attention on it in our research. We prefer to research anomalous behavior: the fraudulent, the criminal, and the immoral, but also successful behavior. Innocent behavior is far less interesting to us.

Sociologists are just ordinary people. That's why even shattered innocence doesn't catch their attention until it affects them personally. When it comes to taking things for granted in everyday life, sociologists remain remarkably aloof. Ethnomethodologists are the exception.[4] They study how people allow life to simply happen, to themselves and to others. But even this branch of sociology, which is storming ahead in America and England, did not make many inroads in the Netherlands. Apparently we find it too ordinary. Is that because Dutch sociologists themselves are so ordinary? Is that why their primary interest is in the unusual?

Healthy people are like sociologists. They know that illness has its consequences, of course—that illness makes them dependent, on others and sometimes on equipment, and that illness imposes limitations on social intercourse. But the fact that illness also means shattered innocence is not something they realize unless they are forced to experience it themselves, to be ill. Then they find out personally that, from a sociological point of view, sick people suffer from "innocence interrupted." When sickness strikes, it's not only the body that breaks down but the life we take for granted as well.

The Puzzle of Fatigue

Being ill means not being able to do things. People who are sick know this. People who care for the sick, home caregivers, are especially aware of it. They see sick people when they're floundering. People who visit the sick are somewhat less aware of it. The ones who are least aware are hospital caregivers. They see sick people mainly in bed. They don't know what sick people are able to do, so they don't know what they aren't able to do, and they really don't know what they'll never be able to do again. It's that inability to do things that interests healthcare researchers, those who study the "quality of life" of the sick. In their questionnaires, at least, they often ask what the sick are capable of: from "climbing stairs" to "having an erection."

The inability to do things is the outward manifestation of the sick person's limitations. But there's more to this inability than meets the eye. In a world based on ability, inability is an all-encompassing problem. In that world, ability is not just ability; it's also a sign of fitness, of youthfulness, of acquired skills, of status and social position, of prestige and honor, of respectability and good breeding, of being able to join in, and of belonging. Inability is the opposite of all these.

Sometimes not being able to do things dominates a person's clinical picture. In my own research among people with chronic illnesses, one man complained bitterly that he was no longer able to muster the energy to operate his sailboat. The boat had been his life, apparently. His inability ruined his existence. The inability of the sick to do things means that their customary level of social participation is reduced, which has a negative effect on their self-image. The inability to do things interferes with their day-to-day lives.

Not being able to do something can have many causes. Fatigue, for example. Everyone knows the feeling, and usually people understand where it comes from: too little sleep, too much work, or a period of being ill and not yet having fully recovered. This fatigue is a matter of common knowledge: "if you exert energy and don't get enough rest, you get tired." We take this for granted. Everyone has experienced such fatigue. It's part of the rhythm of daily life. It's not unexpected and it doesn't require special attention. It just happens every now and then.

There is no sociology of fatigue, at least not that I'm aware of, probably because it's just too common. But it's because it is common that it deserves the attention of sociologists. What makes it common is that the fatigue is usually understandable, and often it's even taken for granted. If someone says he's tired, we take it for granted that there's a good reason for it.

Although fatigue doesn't have the legitimacy value of sickness, it's generally accepted as a justification for not being able to do things. Because it has that justification potential, many people use fatigue as an excuse. That does not always work, however. Fatigue does have to fit into the whole picture.

That's why unusual fatigue is a problem. Unusual fatigue calls the fatigue itself into question. People with such fatigue are unable to offer an acceptable explanation to themselves or to others. Fatigue without a cause is difficult to accept as a justification for not being able to do things. That is why people suffering from unusual fatigue are relieved by the diagnosis of an illness. Fatigue without a medical name creates problems for them. But simply having a name for their complaint is not enough. It has to be a well-established name. So people with an illness like ME (chronic fatigue syndrome) run into difficulties, which accounts for their passionate appeals to find a cause. But even if fatigue has an illness at its root to explain it, it's still not always ordinary.

* * *

In the case of my illness the fatigue has been different. My fatigue is not ordinary. It's not the natural consequence of something. Suddenly, and without cause, I'm tired. The fatigue pervades my everyday existence. It's not closely linked to my illness, however. There's something inexplicable about it. If my illness makes me tired, why does it come so unexpectedly, so haphazardly?

I still remember my first walk through the park just outside our door. The first hundred meters were fine. Then there was a bench, thank God. Then a little bit further, then the next bench. By the time I got to the fourth bench I was worn out. Our house was on the other side of the canal. But it wasn't just a canal that separated me from my bed. I sat down and I couldn't take another step. Mar went home and came back to the park with the car, loaded me in, and took me home. I fell asleep as soon as my head hit the pillow. At that time I still had an explanation for my fatigue: the first walk.

The walking soon improved, but the fatigue remained. Now, however, it came unannounced, without cause. From one moment to the next I couldn't do a thing; I was glad I could make it to my bed. The more time that elapsed since the operation, the more difficult it was to account for it. The more my normal life returned, the more abnormal my fatigue became.

Unexpected fatigue disrupts the rhythm of the day. It's not just something that happens in the morning after a bad night's sleep. It's not just something that happens in the evening after a long day at work with lots of chores. Sometimes it hits me in the morning at eleven o'clock after only one hour of work, even though the day before I had worked for four hours straight. And sometimes it comes first thing in the morning and stays with me, for the entire day on occasion. But there are other days when I feel inexhaustible, and I get a second wind at eleven-thirty at night. Or I bike from Berg en Dal near Nijmegen to Utrecht in a single day, against the wind, and after five minutes at home I feel completely rested. But the next time I go out for a bike ride I may suddenly find I'm unable to go another inch. "Hunger pangs," the cycling professionals say, but I've just put away an entire meal.

How do you explain it? The people around me were ready and eager to help me figure it out. They said it was the operation, that I'd be tiring easily for a long time to come. I only partially believed this. But when a doctor also told me, "You've had major abdominal surgery, Mr. Nijhof, and there's no way you're going to be able to do everything you want," I was willing to accept it, at least for the time being. Others said I had to "build up my condition." That, too, seemed plausible—for a while. Later I came up with my own possible causes. Did I overdo it at some point? Did I walk too long yesterday? Forgot my salt? Was my digestion out of whack? Did I work too long? Want to do too much? I had to come up with new theories for my unusual fatigue, theories that would help me start accepting my fatigue as normal again, the way I used to. I wanted my fatigue to be "natural."

And not only for myself. The fatigue also had to be comprehensible to the people around me. They were well-meaning, helpful people. They kept coming up with their own new explanations. "You're doing too much," and "there's too much going on inside your head." And then there were "the illness," "the complications," "the medicines," "the infection," and on top of that the "internal wounds" that "probably hadn't entirely healed yet." And there was my "back pain" and the fact that I was "sleeping badly" because of it. And wasn't there also the "fear of metastasis"? I was inundated with reasons for my fatigue, so many that if they were all true I'd never be fatigue-free again.

While all this was going on, I had no choice but to start accepting my new fatigue as normal. I had to learn how to be tired all over again. I had to learn to apply new explanations to my fatigue, and in so doing to start taking the fatigue for granted again. That meant believing in the fatigue theories. The simplest and most plausible was the one supplied by the doctors. According to that theory, my operation had left me with a "smaller gas tank," and that the "warning light" had become defective. So I would suddenly run out of fuel sooner than expected, and therefore I'd have to lie down sooner than expected. The myth of the previous day was also useful. Whenever I got tired, I'd tell myself that yesterday I must have done something unusual. Most of the time I actually found something. "Worked too long yesterday." "That walk was all uphill." Thus the fatigue was explained and life could go on. It's easy to prove your own theories, but I never believed them entirely. Was there really nothing else? It occurred to me, however, that "thinking there might be something else" would only tire me out, so I turned my thoughts elsewhere.

Evidently I found it difficult to see my fatigue as normal. It refused to become part of my life. Maybe I had to give into the people who said it was just a matter of getting older. Maybe a doctor would appear with impressive professional credentials who would take some far-fetched explanation and make it normal for me. Or is finding an acceptable theory of fatigue still something I have to do on my own?

I don't think it will ever come to that. It's not that there will never be any plausible explanations, but those explanations will never turn fatigue into something normal. Coming up with a theory does not make it part of normal life. The culture I live in does not offer me any self-evident explanations, and the culture that I myself constitute is not self-evident. So my fatigue remains unusual. My fatigue will have to learn to live with unusualness.

And if I were to succeed, then my fatigue would have to be acceptable to others. Sometimes I used to imagine that people were thinking, "Tired already? But yesterday he was so spry." The people around me had to learn to live with my fatigue just as I did, and that is difficult. We need a corresponding theory for that, one that is especially suited to unusual fatigue. Accepting something as normal is not easily acquired. On top of everything else, fatigue is tedious for others. And tediousness will never be normal.

* * *

Fatigue means not being able to do things, but that's a different not-being-able-to-do-things than medical research has come up with. Fatigue is not only not being able to do things. Fatigue is also a matter of breaking through the social game of taking things for granted. Unaccountable fatigue is contrary to the nature of the social. If there is no explanation for it, then fatigue becomes irritating behavior.

The fatigue of the sick is often unusual fatigue, fatigue that comes on unexpectedly and refuses to behave in an ordinary way. So the problem with the fatigue of the sick isn't that things don't get done. The fatigue becomes problematic if it isn't something we can take for granted, if it comes and goes at will. The problem faced by such sick people is that their fatigue is not natural.

In addition, fatigue cannot be seen. You *feel* it more than anything else. Fatigue does manifest itself, but not in terms of demonstrable behavior—in lethargy, for example, or slowness, or absentmindedness. Fatigue is hidden, hence the frequent reaction, "Oh, come on now!" What do they know?

So the fatigue of the sick is not an individual problem. Fatigue is disconcerting to the sick and to the people around them. Both get caught up in this "puzzle of fatigue." Many "quality of life" researchers, however, think only in individual terms, even sociologists. They examine the limitations and the fatigue of sick people alone and not of their social networks. But sickness imposes limitations on those networks just as it does on the sick themselves.

Fatigue marks out a place in society in which people have trouble finding their bearings. Fatigue is without culture, so it's also without traffic regulations. Fatigue is noninstitutionalized, to use a fancy word. As a result, tired people and their relations have to make their own way. They have to come up with their own rules of the road and deem them acceptable. They have to agree on the causes and on the fatigue that results. This requires a great deal of negotiation. Fatigue calls for people with social skills.

Notes

1. This is what medical sociologists who are "conversation analysts" do. They study the verbal interactions between physicians and patients. See for example, Maynard (1992) and Ten Have (1995).
2. For the early spotting of such crises by a psychiatrist, see Caplan (1964: 34–55).
3. "Naturalness" is not a given aspect of social life, as we read in sociological treatments of the process of "naturalization" (Nijhof 1998).
4. Ethnomethodologists have turned "the ordinary" into a field of research. It is focused on studying how people use ordinary ("ethno") means to fashion everyday life and to explain it at the same time. For standard works from this tradition, see Garfinkel (1967) and Heritage (1984).

References

Caplan, G. 1964. *Principles of Preventive Psychiatry*. London: Tavistock.

Garfinkel, H. 1967. *Studies in Ethnomethodology*. Englewood Cliffs: Prentice-Hall.

Heritage, J. 1984. *Garfinkel and Ethnomethodology*. Cambridge: Polity Press.

Lyons, R., et al. 1995. *Relationships in Chronic Illness and Disability*. Thousand Oaks: Sage.

Maynard, D. 1992. On Clinicians Co-implicating Recipients' Perspective in the Delivery of Diagnostic News. In *Talk at Work: Interaction in Institutional Settings*, ed. P. Drew & J. Heritage, 331–358. Cambridge: Cambridge University Press.

Nijhof, G. 1998. Naming as Naturalization in the Medical Encounter. *Journal of Pragmatics* 30: 735–753.

Parsons, T. 1952. *The Social System*. London: Tavistock.

Scheff, T. 1984. *Being Mentally Ill: A Sociological Theory*. Chicago: Aldine.

Taylor, K. 1988. Telling Bad News: Physicians and the Disclosure of Undesirable Information. *Sociology of Health & Illness* 10 (2): 109–132.

Ten Have, P. 1995. Disposal Negotiations in General Practice Consultations. In *The Discourse of Negotiation*, ed. A. Firth, 319–344. Oxford: Pergamon.

CHAPTER 3

Incantation

Abstract Serious sickness drives the patient to look for magical ways to expel anxiety. One such "incantation" is what I call "techno-security," my trust in the complex medical apparatuses that surrounded me in the Intensive Care Unit and my fright when I was disconnected from them and returned to the ward. It was very different from what I had been reading with regard to medical technology from my sociology colleagues. Another incantation was my attempt to "exorcize" death by working extra hard to keep from thinking of death. An impossible effort, of course.

Keywords Techno-security · Machines · ICU · Time · Panic

Techno-Security

Sociologists who write but don't do research are often moralists. Such moralists tend to be suspicious of technology. They fear control and dependency, as well as loss of autonomy. They see technology as an anonymous power that takes the place of personal care—by doctors, for instance. Seldom have I read about the confidence that machines provide, about "technological peace of mind."

Sociologists who do conduct research see more. They see that technology sometimes offers sick people more options than doctors can provide (Locker and Kaufert 1988; Kaufert and Locker 1990).

G. Nijhof, *Sickness Work*,
https://doi.org/10.1007/978-981-13-0326-5_3

They see that machines reduce dependencies, although they sometimes give rise to new ones. Doctors may tell their kidney patients that dialysis is a "do-it-yourself" procedure, but they still exercise control—over both the machine and the patients. These doctors say "democracy" but do "domination," albeit professional domination (Silverman 1987: 205–232; Alexander 1981) "So *you* do it yourself then," their patients mutter under their breath. Machines are more unambiguous in their behavior. When they offer options to a sick person, they don't insist on assuming responsibility.

* * *

After my operation I was surrounded by machines for quite some time. Later a whole system of tubes and bags was devised for me which the nurses and I managed together, sometimes in consultation. At a certain point my body began to feel like a machine as well.

I woke up with the machines in the intensive care unit, to a very regular succession of ticks and hisses. For a moment I wondered, "What would happen to me if one of them broke down, or if it just stopped working without anyone taking notice?" Soon, however, I saw the people around me. They spoke to me in a friendly way, but they also kept casting strange glances at something hanging over my head. Later on I realized that these must be various meters that showed how my body was functioning. After the initial agitation I found that the machines were making me feel secure. I was being looked after not only by people but also by machines. I could start exploring my surroundings without anxiety.

For I needed to start exploring. I didn't know where I was. Nor did I know why I was there, or how long I had been there, or how long I had to stay. The staff were very friendly, but they wouldn't tell me what I was there for. I think they thought I already knew. Or maybe not even that. They seemed to take it as a matter of course that I knew what was going on. That's why they thought that anybody would know it was the intensive care unit, or the ICU, which is what you have to learn to call it. And they seemed to take it entirely for granted that I knew I had been operated on. I still remember that it took a while for this fact to dawn on me. "They must have cut into my abdomen," I said to myself. But I didn't feel anything there, and my arms were all hooked up to the machines so I couldn't use them to find out. I didn't spend much time thinking, though. I kept dozing off.

Later on I really started wondering about my surroundings. The main thing I saw was the ceiling, but I heard several different voices. "Squeeze my hand," I was told. Whatever could that mean? I had never heard people say such a thing so many times before. "Look at me" was something else I heard with quite some regularity. And then there was all that shouting of numbers. And lots of phone calls. Right up close to me. I knew it was a hospital but I had never heard of a hospital with a Talking Ward.

Then this man in white kept coming to my bed. He talked to me, but he didn't expect me to respond. Even when I didn't say anything he was still very friendly. He started tinkering with my machines more and more. He seemed very competent, so later on I called him doctor. He told me he was a nurse. And then I went back to sleep. When I woke up there was the man again. He said everything was fine, and that maybe this afternoon I could move to the regular ward. No, thank you, I said to myself. I'm doing fine here. "Do they have machines there, too?" He gave me a friendly laugh. "Why should I give up the security of having this man around?" I wondered.

After a great deal more tinkering I was finally disconnected from the machines and wheeled to my ward. As soon as I got there another nurse bounded up to me. Someone who liked machines. After working on them for an hour he broke for lunch and another nurse took over the mechanical construction. "I hope she knows what she's doing," I said to myself. She seemed a bit less skilled. Did she know what my situation was? I watched with fear and trembling. After an hour she looked with satisfaction at me and at the machines, which I could hear behind me, and at the tubes and bags hanging all around. I looked at it all with suspicion. Were all the connections secure? Were the right amounts passing through the tubes? What worried me the most was a sharp, irregular noise coming from a machine behind me: "trr-trr-trr-pss-tak-trr-trr-trr-pss-tak." None of my machines in the intensive care unit made that sound. With every screech the machine's vulnerability forced itself upon me. It sounded as if it were about to become unglued. I complained about the sound. "Yes," said the nurse, "we have better equipment in the ICU." This admission did not calm me down.

I tried to get used to it. I had no choice. I tried to let the strange rhythm lull me to sleep, but it didn't work. There was something unnatural about the sound, I thought. "Typical techie problem," I said to myself. "Failing to realize that you have to be able to sleep with machines, too."

But finally I got used to them. After a few days the IV drip that ran into my neck was disconnected. I was not pleased. "Is my body strong enough to go it alone?" I wondered. The disconnections proceeded apace. During the doctors' rounds the discussions seemed mainly to be focused on which machines I could be weaned from. I was forced to take my leave from them one by one. Sometimes I didn't even know the machine had been there in the first place. There had been a tube running through my penis that I hadn't even noticed. You can leave that one alone, I thought. But I had to let them all go. What remained were the drains. A number of tubes ran out of my body and various things were being collected in bags along the side of the bed. One was a bag for urine, one for discharge from the wound, and on my belly there was a bag for my feces. The nurses had become stevedores for unloading my cargo.

The tubes and their containers also gave me a sense of security. You could see that something was coming out and you could also see how much. I was under control. And because of all that discharging my organs didn't necessarily have to do any work, I thought. The waste products seemed to drain by themselves, even without the help of the organs.

The beauty of the machines became apparent when it was decided that my body had to start functioning on its own: urinating, to begin with. One day later it was clear that my bladder wasn't yet ready. Another catheter was inserted. After a while another attempt was made, again without success. Finally it was decided to introduce a tube through my stomach wall, something else with a gorgeous name that everyone knew but me: "suprapubic catheter." Apparently that was the accepted technology, so I trusted it. Back to the operating room. I was met by a team, ready to put me under with their needle and their jokes and to insert a suprapubic catheter. The tube hurt for days, but I felt reassured. A machine had taken over the functions of a part of my body. I longed for more, for more security, certainly with all those people around me who were keeping things under control.

The equipment made me start thinking about my body in terms of a machine. I now saw my intestines as a drainage canal that could become obstructed, like the damming up of the River Maas. My urinary tract had become an oil refinery. Production units, reservoirs, a system of wires and pipes: that's how it looked to me, something I could picture from having lived near the Botlek, the oil region outside

Rotterdam. Fecal production was a waste disposal unit. Some products in the unit burned better than others. Certain materials had to be added to promote incineration. I found that out when the unit began having problems and all the materials went the wrong way and stayed there for quite some time. Finally they were drained off in vast quantities by means of a tube.

The machines calmed me down. I must have thought I had become just like them: reparable if anything broke down, replaceable if one of them refused to work. And you can see them, so you can monitor them. With the body it's always a guessing game. "How often do you urinate per day?" one doctor asked me. I told him I had never counted, much to his surprise. With the machines and their meters that was no longer necessary. I didn't have to worry about my body anymore. For everything that went wrong in my body there would be a machine to replace it. That was my fantasy. I was entirely satisfied with my machines.

That feeling was reinforced by the trouble I kept having every time one of them was disconnected. A drain for my abscess was disconnected—but too soon, as it turned out. The suprapubic catheter was removed, but my bladder didn't want to work. When an operation was also performed on my prostate it was discovered that my urethra was blocked, and I had to rely on the simplest of all machines, a little tube. At that point I no longer trusted my body very much. It felt second-rate, like something made by hand before the age of automation.

By regarding my body as a system of tubes that could only work efficiently when hooked up to machines, I held death at bay. Machines only have to be adjusted and, in the most extreme cases, replaced in order to sustain life. But the more machines I had to part with, the more I feared death.

* * *

Machines are mainly understood as things outside the human body. But it is possible for machines to become part of our bodies, our "own." This is disturbing for people who fear that a machine might break down unnoticed. But if that possibility can be addressed and anticipated, then machines can bring the peace of mind that comes with having control.

As the control increases, however, we become more anxious about the things that are not yet being controlled. And that is the tragedy of progress. One man's progress is another man's setback.

Beating Death

We don't think about sickness and death in our day-to-day lives. That's why we take life for granted. It has its tomorrow and its day after tomorrow. We talk about next year without blinking an eye. Even thinking about longer periods doesn't unsettle us. We think far into the future, about what has yet to be done, we make plans and think about our pensions and about the pleasant things we're going to do when we retire. We think quite matter-of-factly in the long term, and there's no room in that everyday matter-of-factness for anxiety about tomorrow, no need for short-term thinking.

Illness breaks through that matter-of-factness. Illness makes life unstable, and makes its course unpredictable. Sick people become insecure about how much time they've got left, and that insecurity doesn't go away when the illness has passed. Illness influences our sense of time.

Only some sociologists regard time as important. They call attention to "changes" in time and even speak of "long-term processes." Sociologists who think in shorter terms speak of "careers" and "walks of life." And even shorter terms have to do with "reactions," such as "processing" and "adaptation."

But for many sociologists time plays almost no role at all. They describe social phenomena as if they were timeless and not subject to change, as if the social world they describe just "is." This is not because these sociologists don't think time is important in their particular field. It is because they are ordinary people, too, and they are part of the ordinary world of matter-of-factness. In that world, time may be "money," but the fact that there *is* time is simply normal. That world is organized in such a way that tomorrow is taken for granted. No one ever calls up in the morning to find out if their place of work still exists. The world will just keep on turning, or so we think. Time as we experience it rarely means "finitude." Under ordinary circumstances, in ordinary lives, continued existence is taken for granted. Only the exceptional few talk about their fear of not surviving tomorrow. We regard life as natural. We may run short of time, but it's really unlimited—at least that's how we usually see it. We live in the unconscious certainty of a tomorrow. Unconsciously there is always time. Time has become part of nature: it's there and it's always going to be there, as if it were natural. If time weren't money, we'd just have to "fritter it away."

Sociologists study the experience of time mainly in exceptional situations, when the unconscious is breached: when people in a crisis lose their sense of time, or when they become anxious about what the future holds, or when their future is threatened in the event of disasters and catastrophes, or when they find themselves in situations of stress and nervous exhaustion, when they're constantly plagued by the idea of being short of time. But we always study these situations as exceptional, as unconventional, as moments in which our feeling that "time is ordinary" has been shattered.

But even this kind of time research is rare when it comes to the sick. When the experience of time is investigated in relation to illness, it is usually as the cause of illness and not as its consequence. The stress of feeling harried, of deadlines, and of excessive demands has indeed been a topic of research on the possible causes of health problems. But the impact of illness on the experience of time is a relatively unexplored research domain.

* * *

What is the meaning of life when death threatens, when it's no longer possible to take life for granted? First, for me, there was crisis and panic. Now that I could no longer count on life as a foregone conclusion, I didn't know what to do. Panic. Like people in a burning house who carry their eggs out and leave their valuables behind, I had lost sight of life's priorities. I was adrift. When I heard I had cancer I just wandered through the house. I didn't know why I was upstairs or down. Then came the attempt to get a grip on life. In my case the best way to do that was by means of obsessive–compulsive behavior. Doing the same thing over and over again gave me a sense of order, especially if I succeeded in actually bringing order about. For nights on end I would arrange the books on the shelves in my study. I had just moved, so there was no lack of work to be done. Then came the external organization. The treatment began. For a long time I didn't have to look after myself at all. Other people planned my life for me. Being under treatment provided me with a well-regulated existence. Doctors and nurses took on a great deal of the work themselves, so it was out of my hands. All my thinking about time in my life was superseded by the urgency of the treatment. There was a lot to do, and no escaping it. I was sick and my life was being lived for me, and that was good. The precariousness of my existence simply disappeared beneath all the attention and scheduled meddling. I was sick and I pulled myself together, but now as a sick person.

But soon there were more questions, and with them came insecurity. How do I go on? And how much longer have I got? At that point it hit me: my sense that life was something you took for granted had been undermined. Only later did I realize that once again I had come up with my own strategy for dealing with this. I've never been a laid-back person, but since becoming sick I've had the feeling that I am being hounded. I don't allow myself any time for rubbish and I'm constantly planning new things: do this, take care of that, just one more book.

I was already working on a book, but as soon as I got sick another one popped into my head. "I think I'd be reading a comic book," my surgeon remarked when he happened to see me the day before the operation sitting on a bench in a corridor of the hospital with part of my book manuscript in my hand. Five days after my operation I was back at it, editing the text—or at least that's what I thought: I added the occasional comma. I wasn't able to concentrate on other people's books; after three sentences I had completely lost the gist. But I didn't have to understand my own texts. All I had to do was tinker with them. This has been going on for quite some time now. For months after my operation I worked on my books, which had now become many. At first I worked for short periods: minutes at the most, a quarter of an hour, followed by hours of rest. Very slowly things picked up. By three hours of work I found myself with a daily routine. But I took on more and more. Now that I'm writing this book, I've given myself two weeks to complete it. And it didn't stop there. In the year of my illness I published articles in several academic journals. In fact they had been written before I became ill, but they required radical rewriting. For the journals' editors, being sick wasn't a factor; they simply asked if the article could be ready within four weeks. I shut my mouth and did the work.

Why all that fuss about something that for some time had seemed to be the end of my life? Why that pressure to get to work?

I had once heard that after a serious illness people just wanted to look at the flowers, or read from the classics, or listen quietly to ancient music. None of that for me. Totally uninterested. For months my bed was right next to our bookcases, the classics all within reach, but I didn't touch a single one. I don't even remember what I was lying next to. I just kept tinkering endlessly with the umpteenth version of umpteen texts. Working on your own book is a good way to "beat sickness." It was work that took me to another world and separated me from the illness, there in my own bed and with my own book. My head was momentarily free of the disease.

Doing sociology kept me from losing it completely. But it wasn't just sociology that kept me going. There was also the unarticulated realization that it could all be over soon. The sense of unlimited time was gone, the feeling that time would always be there. That feeling evaporated when I became ill. I had to hurry up.

One aspect of this was narcissism, of course: the desire to mean something, to be remembered, not to take any unwritten ideas with me to the grave, to be read. But it felt as if there was more.

First of all, my head was too tired for anything other than myself. I had never realized that before, that the head is also part of the body. Whenever I thought of fatigue I thought about the rest of my body but never my brain. My legs could refuse to go another step, but I rarely thought my brain would behave that way. Apparently I just took it for granted that my brain was always in a state of readiness. Whenever I went to the bathroom during my illness, it tired me out so completely that I had to rest for an hour. When it came to reading a book by Bourdieu, however, I was sure I could read at the same speed that I did before. That proved to be an illusion. It was just like my trips to the bathroom: slow, with stops and new starts. The brain, as it turns out, is just part of the body.

Reading my own work was far less trouble, mainly because it was limited to commas and periods, and the most I had to do was move words around. I wasn't reading, I was looking, because I already knew what was there.

But there was more. There was also the "self-occupation": keeping myself busy, doing things that had nothing to do with my illness. Being sick forces this on you anyway. Not only is sickness highly labor-intensive, but it also requires a great deal of attention. Other people are always talking to you about it. In the hospital you don't get any rest at all. First the nurse comes to take your blood, then the dietician comes to talk about food, then there's the lady with the books, then your surgeon who wants to know how it's going, then the woman with the beverages asking what you want to drink, then the meal lady who wants you to write down what you think you're going to want for breakfast, lunch, and supper; and on top of that there are the ward physicians and the residents and mainly the nurses who spot all kinds of problems and come up with lots of solutions to keep their sick people busy. And then there's the visitor who wants to know how you and your illness are doing. It's not easy for sick people to think about their illness.

Sociology is a good field to be in for beating sickness. All a sociologist needs are a pair of eyes, a hand that works, a pen, and some paper. We really are blessed. Chemists need a laboratory. Bricklayers, if they're lucky, can stare out the hospital window and look at other people's work, but that's it. Most of them are stuck with nothing to do at all except ask the nurses questions, talk with their fellow patients, and wait for visitors. They might don a headset or pick up a book to shut out the world, or they might connect to the world by means of their phone. But in most cases it's clear that being sick is not what their lives are all about. They start brooding. Writing-based scientists like me, on the other hand, can get to work anywhere, anytime, with nothing but a piece of paper. There's nothing to keep sick sociologists from practicing their trade. All they have to do to conduct their research is look around them. Their profession keeps their mind off their maladies.

But mostly I worked from an unwillingness to call it quits, to keep from having to admit that this might be the end. Writing was my way of fighting off thoughts about death, of dispelling the idea that the prospect of death could silence me, of acting as if death had no dominion. Writing was "beating death." I wrote my way across the border between death and life. To shake my fist at death: that's why I wrote.

* * *

The people we interview as medical sociologists seldom talk about death. But because we, too, are human beings, we also never ask about it. Anthropologists seem to have a bit more nerve. In the Netherlands, Robert Pool and Anne-Mei The closely observed how dying people, their doctors, and their families deal with the fear of death and last requests. Medical sociologists limit themselves mainly to talking about what usually precedes death: illness, and then preferably based on impersonal questionnaires.

But when a medical sociologist himself becomes ill, there's almost no getting around it. He can start writing, of course, but the mind doesn't let itself be restrained so easily. It slips in between and behind other ideas and starts thinking about death. Such a sociologist must relate to life in the short term. He can no longer pretend death isn't there. When death breathes down your neck, it worms its way into your life. Some people look at the little animals and the flowers and say they're enjoying whatever has been left to them. Others become restless, which sometimes leads to an unrestrained impulse to work as long as they can. "Precarious existence": that might serve as the basis of an excellent sociological study. The threat of death is a very good peephole for observing what illness can do to life.

The threat of death does not leave people unfazed. They do something about it. What they do about it usually isn't much different than what they have always done. A human being is not quick to change. He's gone to a lot of trouble to become the way he is, and if his behavior isn't deliberately acquired, at least it's what he's become accustomed to. It's with that baggage that he goes to face the crisis of his illness.

Sick people don't just *become* limited in their behavior, they also limit themselves. They do that to avoid the precariousness of their own existence. They beat time, sickness, and death. What they seem to prefer is to be occupied by something other than themselves. But in doing so they often fall back on themselves, doing what they have taught themselves to do, what they are used to doing. This makes sick people somewhat monomaniacal. It seems to me that the most disturbing illnesses are those that keep people from doing what they were accustomed to doing. The most troublesome sick people are those who can no longer live their normal lives.

References

Alexander, L. 1981. The Double-Bind Between Dialysis Patients and Their Health Practitioners. In *The Relevance of Social Science for Medicine*, ed. L. Eisenberg and A. Kleinman, 307–329. Dordrecht, Boston, and London: Reidel.

Kaufert, J., and D. Locker. 1990. Rehabilitation Ideology and Respiratory Support Technology. *Social Science and Medicine* 30 (8): 867–877.

Locker, D., and J. Kaufert. 1988. The Breath of Life: Medical Technology and the Careers of People with Post-respiratory Poliomyelitis. *Sociology of Health & Illness* 10 (1): 23–40.

Silverman, D. 1987. *Communication and Medical Practice: Social Relations in the Clinic*. London: Sage.

CHAPTER 4

Collective Disruption

Abstract When it comes to illness we think mainly of the individual who is directly affected. In doing so, we deny not only our profession but also those who are close to the sick person. My wife and children were also suffering. Illness is a collective experience. Moreover, sociologists claim that sick people are subject to network shrinkage, but shrinkage does not mean loss alone. I discovered that other people grew closer to me, and I to them. Sickness makes one dependent, but others also become dependent on the sick person.

Keywords Collective illness · Network · Dependency

Collective Illness

Illness and being ill is mainly an individual matter—at least that's how the thinking goes in our culture. And health care is organized around that culture. Illness is something that happens to individuals, even though the actual situation can often be quite different. Cold and flu occur in collectives. AIDS is usually connected with contamination by others. Psychic disorders are nearly always relational phenomena.

But hospital beds are single beds, and the only people occupying them are the sick, not their "neighbors." The people being cared for in those beds are referred to in individualistic terms. And once they have arrived at the hospital they are called "patients."

G. Nijhof, *Sickness Work*,
https://doi.org/10.1007/978-981-13-0326-5_4

But most of these patients are part of a network of people, usually people who are closely related, people who are involved in each other's lives in complex dependencies. Health care, with its individualistic concepts, infringes on these relationships.

* * *

I was ill and I underwent an operation, but it was my partner who had to deal with the consequences, especially in the beginning. I was flat on my back, but she did all the footwork. My children also organized their working hours to be with me. I just looked idly by from my sickbed. My life as a sick person was only apparently individualistic.

The work that my malady required of me every day did not take place in the inhabited world. Elaborate visits to the bathroom twelve times a day. Cleaning all my tube hook-ups. Changing bandages. Cleaning the colostomy bag and replacing it on time. That meant tidying things up, cutting things to size, treating irritated skin. And then cleansing the opening of the suprapubic catheter with iodine and getting rid of the pus from my internal infection. Changing my clothes when, once again, I became soaked with sweat. Making sure I ingested enough salt. All that took place in almost complete isolation. I was too busy to give much thought to pleasantries beyond my individual life as a sick person. I had to make sure I got through my daily program.

Books were sent to me from outside, but they ended up on the "unread" pile. Museums held no interest for me. I gave no thought to new clothes, nor did I devote any attention to receiving visitors. I didn't fantasize about vacations. I didn't even know what month it was.

But this wasn't at all true for Mar. The things we did together suddenly ceased to exist. Illness ruins not only your daily existence but also your daily coexistence.

If I didn't think about that life, Mar did it for me. But even a vacation never got beyond the thinking stage. Thinking about a vacation was something she actually enjoyed because it was a way to remember our old life, of going out together, away from "our" illness.

I was sick, and my illness kept me so busy that I took a limited life for granted. I couldn't think about anything else. But Mar was limited only by me. She didn't see this limitation as unavoidable and normal. All the rest of her life proceeded as usual: her work, our house, and the day-to-day task of caring for me. That's why the idea of vacation kept cropping up, as it does with all ordinary people.

The only place we could travel to was in her head: to cities and faraway countries, as we were used to doing. She told me what she was thinking about. All I could think about, for the time being, was the here and now. For her, in "a world of partners," going on vacation with someone else was not an option. All Mar could do was to get through her vacation time "alone" with me, in an empty country, without friends and acquaintances. And whatever friends there were had their own vacation. A short bicycle trip, a family visit, a day out to Amsterdam, buying plants for the garden: it made her vacation without going anywhere that much more solitary.

It wasn't the usual conflict of one wants this, the other wants that. Now it was one wanting something and the other not even thinking about wanting. That is hurtful for the person who wants, although I, too, felt passed over. "You know how difficult things still are for me." A battle of misunderstandings. Talking about it led to inextricable conflict. "I want to go away." "For the time being I can't do anything." "How about buying a travel guide to Jordan?" "If you think you need it."

Sometimes there was a quarrel. With everything we said we were at cross purposes. Finally, Mar was forced to resign herself to the situation. There was no country she could travel to with me.

Our first days out together were a real breakthrough. We were happy to find a small guest room in an old farmhouse in a little village. That evening we ate out for the first time. Back home the next day. That was about all I could manage. I said I was tired when we got back home after a long journey. "We've took a few wrong turns," said Mar.

But no matter what Mar did, she was not allowed to take part in the quality-of-life studies that I participated in during my illness. Of all the questionnaires that were put in front of me when I was sick, not a single one of them was about her, let alone personally addressed to her. Even my fellow sociologists focused their attention on me alone during their research visits. Almost none of my visitors asked about the people I was living with. Almost none of them asked about my partner. The two who did were sociologists who were studying interaction.

* * *

Illness exists, and medical sociologists conduct research on how illness impacts the lives of the sick and of others. These sociologists see that the sick are often able to do less than the healthy and that they often feel differently as well. In their quality-of-life studies, sociologists try to determine which activities sick people are unable or less able to do, and sometimes whether they are unhappy or not. They may also study sick people's contacts, their networks, and they usually find that these networks tend to shrink, which can lead to isolation and loneliness.

The partners of sick people are scarcely included in this research. I forgot about the partners in my own research as well. I noticed that when we asked people with Parkinson's disease for their life stories we were frequently confronted with the story of a "we." "That's how we do it." When we asked for the life stories of the sick, what we often got were collective stories. "I" quickly became "we," "my illness" became "our problem." The sickness work was a collective endeavor. Sometimes the life story itself was told collectively, and the storyteller became a collective. And sometimes the story was even told by the partner, speaking on behalf of "us."

It's a shameful experience for a sociologist, who knows that his profession is all about interactions and relationships but who interviews mainly "individuals" in practice. And it was cold comfort to learn that I was not alone with my shame. Many of my fellow sociologists have adopted the individual interview as their standard method.

I actually knew that the sick and their partners often operate as a collective. I learned it from my literature on people with chronic illnesses. Strauss and Corbin wrote about the work done by people who are involved in the lives of the sick. That work forms the basis of the relationships that develop between them. But what remained largely uninvestigated was how relationships involving the sick become troubled, how people are drawn together by illness struggle to redefine their relationship.

Almost all medical sociologists are just as prone to individualizing their subjects as the healthcare system we research. Although we are the ones who disclose the information, we are just as subject to the domination of medical discourse as anyone else. So when it comes to illness we think mainly of the individuals whom the illness is affecting physiologically. In doing so we deny not only our profession but also those for whom illness is a collective undertaking.

Networks Lost and Found

Medical sociologists are often pessimists. All we tend to see are problems. And the research done on those problems leads to yet more problems. We're like the medical practitioners, steaming up the waterway of "illness" and "devastation." Seen in this way, illness is nothing but suffering and loss and must be fought against without restraint. But sick people also experience many good things—in their networks, for example.

Over the past ten years, sociologists have said that the chronically ill are subject to "network shrinkage" and "dependence." De Swaan (1990) writes that long-term illness, especially illnesses that deteriorate over time, make the patient more dependent on the people around them, often more and more dependent on fewer and fewer people. Research has shown that this is indeed the case. Yet illness does not mean network shrinkage alone. Nor does network shrinkage mean loss and dependence alone.

* * *

My world quickly grew smaller. It wasn't only my professional network that shrank, and that of my friends and acquaintances. They were already minimal in my case. For me the primary loss was my daily exposure to people: people from other parts of the world, fellow passengers in the bus and train, the coffee lady at the station, the people from the cafe where I occasionally stopped to have something to drink, and—and even more anonymous—the people who filled the streets. And then there were the little daily indications of life in the world: a smile, a silent greeting, a sign of recognition, a bit of cursory flirting, a familiar face, a couple watching out for each other. People I saw biking past my house early in the morning, wearing clothes that marked their differences in status and rank: the earliest were the manual laborers in old clothing, the last were the intellectuals with no clock to punch, and in between, at ten minutes before the hour and the half-an-hour, were the secretaries, typists, sales personnel, and employees, neatly dressed and clearly afraid of being late. That was the everyday network that I saw on my journey through life as a sick person. I exchanged no words with them, but they were the cement of my community. My existence as a seriously sick person is much more anonymous than the term "network" suggests. It can also be found in the slight smile on the tram, the faces of busy people. It was that community cement that suddenly dropped from sight when I became ill.

But new cement was made. Other people grew closer to me, and I to them. Old friends who remembered me. Anonymous people who unexpectedly had something personal to confide. Colleagues who all at once became acquaintances. People who quickly became friends. Girlfriends of Mar who actually were my friends, too, although they didn't always let on.

Being ill has reoriented my social life. What I lost with one I gained with the other. There my world became smaller, here it became greater and more intense. With some people life became colder, with others warmer. Illness is both loss and gain (Von Faber and Van der Geest 2010).

* * *

Illness offers too many perspectives to leave it to people who are preoccupied with destruction, erosion, and doom. Illness is too exciting to make it the exclusive property of doctors and the sociologists who follow them.

Illness should not automatically be written off as something destructive, especially not by medical sociologists. For them, too, illness and infirmity are overwhelmingly understood as sources of trouble and affliction, which in turn are caused by more trouble and affliction. All too often, medical sociologists focus on this bias without giving it a moment's thought. When it comes to illness, we have a tendency to emphasize the misery alone. We mindlessly follow the adage "bad causes bad." Illness only comes from bad things, we believe: alcohol abuse, eating fats, trauma, crisis, stress, deprivation, prolonged misunderstanding, and conflict. According to our hypothesis, the main causes of illness are deficiency and excess. And according to the same sociologists, illness goes on to produce more of the same: calamity, sorrow, anxiety, depression, isolation, loneliness, and obstruction. These, we sociologists argue, are the consequences of illness.

But isn't that being a bit too short-sighted? Illness also has its pleasures. By showing what those pleasures are, sociologists can avoid something that they themselves have advanced: the idea of the domination of medicine and the medical pessimism that comes with it.

The Dependencies of Illness

You aren't sick alone. Without others, illness is impossible to live with. Being ill is a process of creating dependencies, particularly in the case of long-term illness. Consequently, sick people become like children. They turn to others for their food and maintenance. If they want company, others have to come to them. And to find out what's going on outside they are dependent on other people's reports.

* * *

The first person I sought out was Mar, to tell her what had happened to me during the hospital examination. I no longer remember what I did, only that I paced from one end of the house to the other. I didn't dare call her because a phone call would have to go through someone else, her secretary. I would never get past her without stammering. So I walked back and forth through the house until Mar called to hear what I had heard. Minutes later she was home and I was able to cry with her. I saw our life changing. I thought I wasn't going to make it, and if I did, it definitely wouldn't be on my own. For the first time I felt dependent.

Other dependencies quickly followed: with the doctors and their retinue. Right from the beginning, I felt that the dependence was only partial; I knew I couldn't rely on it. "It's operable," the surgeon had said. Did he mean this was a solution to the problem? Or was operating just a stay of execution? Could any surgeon do this? Or did I have to start looking for a specialist? And once I had found him, my doubts remained. Was it possible that he might make a mistake? That he might overlook something? Was my body in a more advanced state than he knew?

Even dealing with the doctors was something I did with Mar. Mar called friends to find the name of a competent surgeon. She was with me when I went to see them. We went together, but Mar "did" the doctor. I gave a brief synopsis of what was going on. I answered his questions, but Mar led the discussion. She went further with her questions than either I or the doctor did. She put my insecurities into words. She didn't let the doctor get away with anything. With me he could play the doctor game, but he couldn't get anything past her. I stayed on the sidelines. Mar covered the field. The doctor recognized that. He asked her about her work, told her about problems he was having with his child—as a sign of good rapport.

Then came the operation and the hospital. The operation was an encroachment on my body, but for Mar it was an encroachment on her life, and the lives of others she loved. My son Piotr and my daughter Eva were at my bedside. All three organized their lives around my illness, and they did it for quite some time. Their outward existence was regulated by visiting hours, and they let it be known that the uncertainties of the illness disturbed them. They made themselves dependent on me, and I on them. I was being ill, but they were living my illness.

After all the emotion, the doctors, and the hospital came the routine of daily life. That demanded plain old work—in and around the bed, first of all. That was when I felt my dependence. In the hospital, help is always institutionalized. It seems quite normal there. But at home it's different. In the morning, a tray filled with all the necessities was placed next to my bed. Each item had a special purpose. Bouillon and ham for the salt. Drinks for the fluid. Pills for the illness. And that was just to get through the morning. In the afternoon, Mar came into bring me new provisions, to do what she thought I needed.

Being sick entails multiple dependencies. Without Mar nothing would have happened. First I needed her to cry with, then for the daily maintenance of body and soul, then for the supervised expeditions in the world around me, then for trips farther afield to get our life back. But I wasn't only dependent on her. Mar had also become dependent on me. She could no longer do anything without factoring me into her calculations. Could she get away, or not? Could she be cheerful, or not? Could she go out to eat with friends? I became the gauge by which she measured so many of her activities. Someone who is sick becomes a millstone around people's necks, a wristwatch on their arm.

But the sick person feels dependent, too. Because I was unaccustomed to being sick I also became insecure. How far could I go with my illness? To what extent could I let the illness make a claim on other people? How much can you demand from someone else? When does demanding become tyranny? When does the illness become an excuse?

* * *

I knew from my medical sociology that sick people become dependent on others, but I did not know that those others also become dependent on the sick. It isn't only the sick who lose their autonomy. "His" people lose theirs, too. But the sick person can't help it.

The others organize their lives around what the sick person is able to do, and especially what he is not able to do. This puts the sick person at an advantage. Often he has no choice, but he also has his illness as an excuse. For the others, however, there is less to be taken for granted. For him or her there is only the culture, and thus the morality, in which caring for the sick is an "appropriate" response. Illness is an imperative phenomenon, and therefore a sick person is, too.

Those who wish to can avoid the pressure of dependence by avoiding the sick person altogether. But for those who are close to him this is not an option. Their dependence is colored by social constraint. Their decision to stay is a moral one.

Constraint is an unwelcome element in the cultural context of the partner relationship. Technically, such a relationship is based on love and availability, "till death do us part." But what happens when the loved one is confronted with the role to which he has pledged himself, that of caregiver in times of need?

Sociology has done little research in this area. The precariousness of healthcare relationships is rarely investigated, probably because people are not eager to discuss it. Usually, they go no further than superficial observations. But in our research among the chronically ill we did find traces of it. There was one partner who left the room at the beginning of an interview, causing the person being interviewed to say, "He always does that now when we start talking about my illness." On the other hand, there was the partner who joined the sick partner in telling a life story in terms of "we." Illness does something to relationships, but what exactly does it do?

References

De Swaan, A. 1990. *The Management of Normality*. London and New York: Routledge.

Von Faber, M., and S. Van der Geest. 2010. Losing and Gaining: About Growing Old 'Successfully' in the Netherlands. In *Contesting Aging and Loss*, ed. J.E. Graham and P.H. Stephenson, 27–45. North York: University of Toronto Press.

CHAPTER 5

Sickness Work

Abstract Sickness means hard work, as the title of this essay has announced. But what does this work entail? Being ill is like entering unknown territory and feeling your way, getting accustomed to the unusual. This is followed by training, learning the rules in this new territory, turning the unusual into "normal." One of the most delicate normalizing lessons was handling my stoma in sometimes awkward circumstances. Next came all kinds of daily chores that fall outside the realm of medical care. I was proud that I developed certain skills in taking care of myself, but they were often too intimate to talk about, let alone to show. Finally, sociology is a discipline of the day. Sociologists usually spend the night sleeping. But for me, as a patient, nighttime was another new territory that I had to struggle with when sleep did not come, as is often the case for many sick people.

Keywords Unknown territory · Training · Stoma · Chores · Sickness skills · Night

Feeling Your Way

Being ill is like entering unknown territory. Not so much in the physical sense, since for sick people, the new aspect is often quite a familiar setting: bed and hospital. That is generally where illness plays itself out. Life there is confined and usually strictly regulated. Sick people cannot

G. Nijhof, *Sickness Work*,
https://doi.org/10.1007/978-981-13-0326-5_5

come and go at will. Their freedom of movement is severely restricted: By the sick person himself, by those who are treating and caring for him, and by the unwritten rules of the hospital.

The realm of unfamiliarity is mainly the social. It isn't only the experience of being ill that is new; it's also the meaning of the illness. What does the illness involve? What will you still be able to do with this illness, and what will you never be able to do again? How far can you push yourself? What might you be able to do again, with practice? And when have you crossed the line and gone too far?

This is an area that seriously sick people usually don't know from experience. And they haven't had the chance to learn very much from other sick people because it's hard to read anything from their behavior. A great deal is hidden, varnished over, or suppressed. Stories about the illness are rarely told. Such stories are not held in high regard, and they're often embarrassing to boot. Acknowledging dependence, mentioning blood and feces are not things people are eager to hear.

But there's also another reason why the sick are so reticent. They don't really know what they can talk about and what they should keep to themselves. And if they do say something, other people don't know what to make of it. "Are they really telling us everything?" Or "is it as bad as they say?" Or "isn't that story a little too rose-colored?"

This erratic transfer of information tends to keep healthy people in the dark. If they ever get sick themselves—if it ever gets that far—they'll just have to find out on their own what being sick is all about.

Sociologically speaking, the regulation and institutionalization of being sick is limited. In their formal existence, sick people have the "role" of the sick person at their disposal. They can adopt this role to show others that their illness also has social ramifications. Once they've taken on this role they can exhibit unconventional behavior, such as not working. If they are officially declared sick, they can legitimately abandon their obligations without feeling distressed. But in their informal existence it's much less clear how far they can go. It's hard for others to know what the sick can rightfully abandon. This makes being sick a matter of "feeling your way."

* * *

Being sick for me was far from just being unable to do something. My problem was mainly not being sure of knowing if a thing was possible, not being sure of knowing whether I could still do what I used to be able to do without having to think about it. This involved a lot of trial and error. I had to sound out my body, assay its possibilities. What was too far, and how far could I go? I kept trying to go farther by expanding the things I was doing.

I was a "cyclist" before my illness. Not a grand-scale cyclist, but one with a racing bike, and with stories about trips I had gone on that I called "death trips" when speaking with the circle of people who were willing to put up with my boasting. Most of these were stories from the past. On my later trips, I got better at judging how far I could go. I knew when I shouldn't do any biking and how I'd feel after sixty miles, and how long after that the trip would take. I knew when to get off and when to really stop. But all that knowledge, acquired by means of injury and disgrace, proved obsolete after I became ill. My knowledge of cycling was in disarray.

At first I couldn't bike at all. Then I wasn't allowed to bike. And when I was allowed, I no longer knew what I could or couldn't do. The first short ride went fine. I was less tired than I expected, and I could keep up with Mar reasonably well. We hardly ever talked about biking, more about what we saw while biking. We had a drink somewhere and then went home. As if everything was back to normal.

But then the idea came up of a bike vacation in the Netherlands. We'd see how far I could go. There were little hotels everywhere, right? What could go wrong? We had made reservations in the first hotel on our route forty-two kilometers from home. We'd take it easy. Give ourselves a whole day to get there. I had packed my salt cookies and my customary drinks. The weather was bad so we took shelter several times, which meant making just as many rest stops. But that didn't occur to me at the time. As long as I came to a stop, consumed some salt, and had a drink. Suddenly I realized that Mar was biking twenty meters ahead of me. I'll catch up, I thought. In the next town, we made our first stop. Baguette with cheese, lots of salt on the tomatoes, coffee, and a big glass of mineral water. I didn't feel like I had biked at all. Twelve more kilometers to go. We did it in nothing flat, although with two compulsory stops: Two ferry rides across a river. As soon as we got to the hotel, I had a cheese sandwich and a glass of milk. Hardly paid any attention to my condition.

The next day we stayed in the hotel. Storm and rain. We did a little biking that afternoon. The dike and surroundings were magnificent, but the biking was hard. It was because of the storm, I told myself. We almost got blown off the dike. But we kept on pedaling for a while.

Stopped to take shelter. More pedaling. Shelter again. Then we decided to ride back. I'd been fantasizing about a cheese sandwich for quite some time. Once again, Mar was biking far ahead of me. No big deal, we were sure to pass a cafe soon enough. A little later I realized that even a cafeteria would be fine. And even later I thought that a pancake house would be sure to have something salty. We circled around for kilometers. Closed. Then I saw a big sign along the road with an arrow pointing to a supermarket. They sell sandwiches there, Mar said. But the arrow was pointing back to where we'd already been, and the hotel was still five kilometers farther on. Biking back to the deserted village might be a mistake, the supermarket there might be closed, too. So we kept on going. I fell even further behind Mar. My legs were refusing to pedal. Finally we made it back to the hotel. A cheese sandwich with a lot of salt shaken on top, something to drink, and after ten minutes, I felt strength returning to my body. "Eat salt and drink on a regular basis," Mar said.

The next day on to Nijmegen, destination: the Ooij polder. We biked along the dike. The wind was at our backs. Full sun. Passed a lovely cafe along the dike. But it seemed a little too early to me. After that not a cafe to be seen. So we headed straight for Nijmegen, which turned out to be farther than I thought. I was behind Mar. Mar kept looking back, coasting. And I kept peering into the distance at what I thought were the outskirts of Nijmegen. First an empty industrial park where there was no cheese to be found. Then suddenly an old working-class district, and almost immediately a deserted cafeteria. We parked our bikes and in we went. A surprised man was behind the counter. Clearly no one had ordered a cheese sandwich from him for quite some time. I needed to sit down, but there were no chairs. There were two outside though, under the eaves. We shoved them around and were able to stay half dry. After fifteen minutes, the cafeteria owner motioned to us. The cheese sandwich was ready. Another tongue-lashing from Mar. "Eat more often and drink more." But how much biking could we do if I had to stop every five kilometers. And was it really five kilometers? How long could I bike without having to forage?

After the sandwich, we continued on to Nijmegen. Stopped there for another sandwich. The hotel was full, so on we went to look for another hotel. I knew a couple from years ago. The first one looked a little down at the heels. Kept searching. There had to be one of those old country hotels somewhere around. On we biked, uphill and down. Suddenly Mar was biking behind me. I didn't feel tired anymore. I wanted to see more hotels. "Keep going," Mar said. Back to an earlier hotel. Stayed there. So I could still bike up hills. Even Mar was worn out. Salt and drink, that's what I needed, I now knew.

That kind of thinking makes a person like me overconfident. The next day another trip? Or straight back home? But wouldn't Utrecht be too far? Let's just go. Laid in six packs of juice, a supply of salty chips, and some more salty sandwiches, and on we went. Once again along the River Waal, but this time on the other side. Wind against us. Showers. Many stops to take shelter. Kept buying salt, drank more drinks. And then things started going well. In Wijk bij Duurstede, after so many hours, I was still fit. Ordered more cheese sandwiches, drank plenty of liquids, and back home within two hours.

By trial and error, I learned this new approach to biking. It was just like long ago when, as a child, I learned which turn was too sharp, which sand was dangerous, how fast you could smash into the curb. Now I was learning it all over again. Not so much how long I could bike, or what was too far, or too ambitious, or what I really ought not to do at all. Now the challenge was to figure out what my body needed when I biked. That was what I had to think about now.

The body is equipped to send you warning signs, but that doesn't mean people always acknowledge them. At first I didn't even detect the signs of energy loss. In the past, if Mar had shot out ahead of me it wouldn't have gone unnoticed. Now I simply didn't pick up on it. Not because I was thinking about something else but because I didn't give it any thought at all. The body overrules the thought processes. It lets you bike slower without your even being aware of it.

When you first go too far, you resolve to do something about it: To eat and drink on a regular basis, not only when you feel you need it. I wasn't used to that. Now, however, it was essential. It was something I learned the hard way. And as long as I did that, everything would be fine—or so I thought. I'll bike just the way I always did, right?

But that assumption is an illusion. You have to work for it: Sensing that you're slowing down, understanding what your body needs, learning to read the signals your new body is sending you. All those signs were translated into schedules: for drink, but especially for salt.

This meant that the things I innocently used to take for granted about biking were gone. I had entered a realm of careful assessment: Of looking around and looking ahead. My life as a cyclist had to be reorganized. But now that has happened, things are not worse than I was used to.

Not only does the capacity of the body change, but the habit of taking it for granted changes, too. New habits have to be acquired, with childish trial and error.

* * *

Being ill has become the province of psychology. That's obvious. When people get ill they tend to retreat into a tight little circle, and they go into hiding within their own psyche. They change from social beings to individuals, people with a couple of relations but mainly with a psyche all their own. That's the way it is in psychology. The social aspects are written off.

The psychologists are right to a certain extent. The social lives of the sick are reduced to the bare minimum: Friends who call, colleagues who tell you not to think about work whatever you do. All that remain are the healthcare body artists followed by psychology's balance artists. This makes illness a psychological risk as well, a problem of processing, of emotions, of escapism and avoidance, of emotional expression and self-reproach, of mood, anxiety, and depression, of psychological well-being, of coping. And one's social life is pushed to the background, behind psychology.

What is left of the sick person's social life, however, is not something to be processed as much as something to be worked on: To be learned and managed, with appropriate arrangements to be negotiated. Strauss and Corbin discovered that work among the chronically ill. They also came up with a general term for it: "trajectory work." Sick people have to be socialized all over again. Much of what they had come to regard as normal now seems more difficult, or impossible, to carry out. They're standing askew on the axis of their former existence, and they keep bumping their head. They have to relearn how to live. Most sick people lost the knack of learning how to live when they became adults and knew how to get on with their lives. That idea has now been taken from them. They have to learn to think like children again. They have to readjust to the life that the possibilities of their body now offers them. This can be psychologically difficult, but it can be learned. So for sick people, there's a lot of work to be done. For them, learning to live is exactly the same as it was when they were children: Going too far and having to be called back, falling down and standing back up, refusing to listen to other people and paying for it, opposing people who have your best interests at heart and admitting you were wrong—that's what brings us further.

So there's a great deal to be learned. As you learn, the new life quickly becomes normal again and you can scarcely remember when it was any different. Sick people don't have to remain children. They can feel their way to a new existence, which brings the peace of mind that comes with habituation. After a while, sick people come to regard more and more of their lives as normal and they learn again to be not sick. Feeling their way is only a phase. That's the beauty of what social life has to offer. You get used to more and more things and take them for granted; they don't stay unusual forever. This is what sociology can offer the sick: The certainty that eventually the things that seemed "different" for so long will become ordinary.

At first glance, being ill seems institutionalized by sociological standards. It seems as if people who are ill know where they stand, what they have to strive for, and what they can expect once they get there. And that is true, on the whole. It's true for their social existence and for their official relationships. But is it also true for their everyday experience of being ill? That is uncertain: Their informal social existence is relatively irregular.

It isn't unusual for sociologists to expect the social to be too orderly. After all, regularity and order is by definition the object of their research. When something is irregular, they jump to the conclusion—sometimes all too quickly—that it simply hasn't been researched yet. Once the research is conducted, the order will soon become apparent. But not everything that is unknown appears well ordered and regulated after having been researched. Being ill, for example, is an area where people have to figure a lot out for themselves in order to find ways of doing things that are acceptable to themselves and to others. They have to explore their new life, test the waters, become inquisitive, and often face rejection. In everyday social life, being ill is a makeshift operation. Sociologically speaking, it's a matter of "feeling your way."

Training

At a certain point, the ordinary human being has learned all there is to learn: He can walk and ride a bike, he eats, defecates, and urinates, he knows how to cross the street and greet people and how to tell time. And once he's learned that, it's as if it all came naturally. Illness means not being able to do many of the things had once been taken for granted. Routine activities have to be unlearned and unusual new ones have to be acquired. If learned behavior falters, something new has to be learned to take its place. This is not without its problems. When something has been routine, it's much more difficult to do the same thing a different way.

Medical sociology is mainly concerned with what people no longer can do when they get sick. It is concerned with lost competence, with roles people can no longer fulfill, with worlds from which they are forced to withdraw, and with the difficulty that this new behavior poses.

This sociology has much less to do with the retraining that sick people engage in, the new skills they must acquire, the solutions they come up with, how they master this new behavior, and how all this novelty once again becomes routine. Medical sociology has very little interest in the inventiveness of the sick. It pays scant attention to their innovative work.

* * *

Sick as I was, I had to learn. What I mostly had to learn was how to be sick, and that didn't happen just like that. Nor did anyone teach me, including the healthcare workers who were involved with me and my illness every day.

A colostomy bag fills up by itself, but it also has to be emptied. How do you do that? "Sit on the toilet and put the bag between your legs," said my colostomy nurse. "And afterwards clean it with a sprayer." But other nurses instructed me to measure the amount in a measuring cup. Those were the nurses I saw most frequently, so that's what I did. But when I no longer had to measure the amount, I could reassure the first nurses. I had put the bag between my legs. That seemed to make them happy. He's mastered the technique, I saw them thinking. But that was only in the hospital, as it turned out. When I got home I started by following the prescribed method. Little by little, however, I developed my own techniques, varying according to the amount, the situation, and the time of day, and by different means. Feces stink at home, too. My sense of smell wasn't very keen, but Mar's was all the better, and other people in my vicinity seemed equally adept. They never said anything, but I suspected that they were quite aware of my odor. I had to come up with something to deal with it.

That was life indoors. I hadn't been outdoors yet. That came later on, and when it did I discovered all the things I had yet to learn: Not only the techniques, but also how to deal with my fear that something might go wrong, with annoying people in public toilets, and with my shame at how much time I took and how much stench I was responsible for.

At first I thought I could only go outdoors if I knew where I was going, if I was sure there was a spacious toilet there, with water and soap and not too many visitors. There were plenty of such places in Utrecht, my hometown. Our regular cafe met all my demands. I could take my time there and calmly get the job done. I even snuck in when necessity called without having bought anything to drink.

I couldn't go anywhere else, or so I thought. But then came Mars's vacation. She wanted to go somewhere else for a change, so during her vacation, we took three short trips. And there I was, waiting in line for the toilet in a crowded tourist cafe. No getting around it. It had to be done. Once I got in, I tried to do everything at top speed. I was fairly successful, narrowly escaping the blunders that my nervousness threatened to cause. But then came the loud rattling of the stall door. The next man in line had lost his patience. First I made an attempt at courtesy: "Sorry, just one more minute." That seemed to calm him somewhat. Then came the shouting. "There are more of us out here, you know!" "We're on vacation, too." Finally I opened the door and there we were, two faces reddened by quite different emotions.

Gradually I taught myself not to let the loudmouths get to me. There aren't very many of them anyway. It's mainly the fear of running into them, and I had to get past the fear. Little by little I began visiting unknown cafes and restaurants almost without thinking about it, and I even ventured to take corner seats in playhouses and movie theaters.

One year later, I was ready for a brief vacation abroad. Cafes were far from abundant, and the same was true of soap and water. So I had to make do with the open air and my own resources. At first I hid in a deserted wood, clumsily maneuvering my pants and underpants in a vertical position and bending over to keep my clothes from getting in the way. At first I didn't always come away unsullied. Nor was I particularly graceful. This was going to require practice and brainwork. But before I got that far, the next urgent need arose. Once again, no one in sight. Mar kept watch, just to be on the safe side. This time the clothes came off. I hung my pants on a tree, underpants beside them. That was better, but it took longer. The next opportunity came after a long walk to the fort of El Pascha on a hilltop in northern Greece. I thought we would be following a mountain road running through an olive grove. I had misjudged. The last kilometers turned out to be asphalt, to make it easier for tourists not encumbered with my particular disability. Because of the paved road, wealthy Greeks had come to live there, Greeks with large, fenced-in gardens. No place to do anything private. And if there was such a place, it would be stampeded by tourists. So up to the ruins we went. There was sure to be a hidden corner there. And there was, but there was also a tourist. Every time I tried to drop my pants he popped up with his camera, in search of beautiful vistas. Finally we discovered a dark corner with only one exit. Cerberus Mar led the way. I went in. Sinister, nervous. More tourists had arrived, Mar announced. She had heard voices as well as scooters. "Hurry up." Down go the pants. Underpants stuck on my wallet. Got the bag opened anyway. The floor was well-trodden sand, so lots of clattering and spattering on my pants. Forgot to bring cleaning wipes. Fiddling with my dropped trousers. Mar warning me that someone was approaching. Pants pulled up. Back outside, checking to make sure nothing had happened. Dirty fingers, shit on my pants, stench in the ruins. Now I really had to think of something.

This should be done sitting down, I realized. If not on a toilet, then on a tree trunk. When we started up the hills, we found the very thing. That was better. Nice and peaceful. Who would think, seeing a man sitting on a tree trunk and seeming to be staring into the distance, of a stinking, bare, defecating rear end? Lower to the ground than vertical, no clatter and no spatter. A few leaves afterward to cover up and no one the wiser, except Mar and me.

That experience made me adventurous and bold. What could go wrong now? At home I decided to go on that bike trip we'd been thinking about for so long, to the river region. There may not be any tree trunks there, but there would be dikes with plenty of undergrowth. And it wasn't a place frequented by tourists, certainly not when a day of rain had been predicted. So off we went to the River Waal with perfect equanimity. On our bikes. Suddenly a full feeling. Hadn't seen anyone for half an hour. So I seated myself at the bottom of the dike. I didn't even ask Mar to be on the lookout. But no sooner had I sat down than I spied two joggers on the dike. They, too, refused to be dissuaded by the rain. Right after them two local girls popped up. They were on their bikes, so they soon reached the joggers. They greeted them cheerfully and passed them by. And because there were so few of us, they didn't give us a moment's thought. A couple of tourists enjoying the view, they must have concluded. The joggers decided that the bench at the top of the dike was the perfect place to stretch their muscles and, as they said to each other, "to get their breathing under control." Interested only in themselves, they too didn't seem to see anything. What could happen to me now? Not only had I developed a technique to deal with my fear, but I had also come up with a way of going about my business that tricked everyone around me.

Recklessly we biked on. I gave little thought to the place or the time, and even less to the general public. Our return along the river dike on the other side proved a bit more difficult, however. The dike was mostly pasture, screened off by fences to keep out passing tourists. There were no bike lanes to separate bikes from cars, either. Motorized locals would tear past unexpectedly. They lived on the outside of the dike. That meant more fences, to mark their property. There were also fences on the inside of the dike to contain the livestock. A driveway to a country estate seemed to offer solution. Mar ducked into the woods, but I didn't think that was necessary. I had seen a tree trunk on the side of the road at the beginning of the driveway. A place to sit. Once I was seated, however, a whole slew of cars drove past. No one honked. I thought I was doing fine. Only when I pulled up my pants did I realize that I had been sitting with my back to a small house with a large window on my side. I didn't see anyone, but that failed to reassure me. Recklessness does not go unpunished. Not only does the fear have to be mastered, but the audacity does, too. I had to arm myself against recklessness.

People with ailments and illnesses have to be trained. Doctors know almost nothing about this. For them it's all about the body, and sometimes only the area being operated on. Nurses know much more. They did these chores for me long before I did them myself. They also taught me a lot, with many demonstrations. They emptied my colostomy bag. They came to my rescue when I once again miscalculated the amount, causing the seal to burst open before I could get to the toilet. Not only did they clean up the mess for me but they also taught me how to reduce the problem. The most important thing they taught me was to regard feces as normal. Cover it over with a towel, without even moving a muscle, and it's gone. But outside the hospital, I had to figure it out for myself.

* * *

Sociologists who deal with illness and disabilities are mainly interested in people's inner workings: How they process their ailments, whether they handle them realistically, whether they recognize the seriousness of their condition without taking refuge in fantasy or denial, and how they cope with their other their disabilities. Coping, too, is often concerned with the inner aspects of illness because sociologists focus on the emotions of the sick person and not on what they actually do.

Most sociologists are not sick, so they don't know what sick people do. They think that sick people feel and think and nothing else: They worry, they feel stress, they feel confused and lonely, they think people have abandoned them. This is what sociologists tend to study, and in doing so they create their own worries.

As a medical sociologist, I had to get sick first to discover what a sick person does. I had to learn to be sick and disabled in order to learn what a sociology of illness should be about. For sick sociologists, there's a lot of work to be done.

Healthcare Chores

Healthcare workers are constantly studying. They're highly trained, and most of them are specialized. We count on their knowledge, which is why we entrust ourselves to them. But because they're specialized, a great deal falls outside their domain. "That's for other people to do." Healthcare workers know a lot of those other people, which is why they so often refer us to them. But as a result they tend to lose track of what's going on. Who has charge of the whole picture? What's being taken care of and what isn't?

What isn't being taken care of is the work that has no name and therefore has no specialism. Every specialism has a name. Work that doesn't have a name doesn't exist for specialists. So there are no specialists for work without a name. It's mainly the sick people themselves who discover what work is yet unnamed and what work is therefore not being done.

There are sociologists who focus on the healthcare organization. They talk about team nursing, lines of communication, teaching organization, and communication networks. Sick people and patients tend to fall outside the scope of their domain because they aren't part of the organization. There are other sociologists—not organizational sociologists—who are concerned with sick people and patients. These sociologists work with "quality of care" and "patient research." But they, too, are looking from a healthcare perspective. They focus mainly on what healthcare workers could do better. What they are already doing is their point of departure.

Then there are sociologists who look further. These are the ones who study the "quality of life" of patients, and especially of ex-patients. They try to find out what these patients still can do and what they no longer can do, what contacts they have lost, how they feel, and where those feelings become problematic. They explore the lives of the sick outside the domain of immediate care. But it is not at all clear how much organized healthcare is influenced by their research findings. When new forms of care are developed, they seem to be the result of market forces, of holes in the market that have been discovered by policymakers and healthcare workers themselves. Patients are not the ones who generate ideas for new care.

* * *

When I actually got sick, I found myself in a hospital before I knew it. My family doctor handed my case over to the specialists without any reaction from me. Specialists have their specialism, not only their official specialism but also frequently something within it. One surgeon will limit himself to vascular surgery and another to liver transplants, and the surgeon who treated me was good in operating on intestinal cancer. My challenge, as soon as I found out what I had, was to find such a specialist. After making a number of phone calls from Mar's network, we finally found him.

The operation went relatively well. The surgeon was able to cut away quite a bit. After some follow-up care, the specialist was finished with me, at least as far as his specialism was concerned. But friendly as he was, he kept showing up at my bedside. A great many decisions had to be made with regard to related issues, especially in the beginning. Could the abdominal drain be removed? What was to be done when the natural flow of urine failed to start up properly? It was my impression that my surgeon wanted all these problems solved as soon as possible. "Typical Doctor A," said one of the nurses whose opinion I highly valued when yet another tube was removed from my body—just a little too soon in his estimation. And sure enough, an infection developed in my abdominal cavity, requiring another specialist. "The best in the house," according to my surgeon. So off we went to see this radiologist: consultation, proposal, and operation. My surgeon was still with me when the operation was over, and he stayed on as my regular doctor. The infection refused to budge. The radiologist lost interest when his operation failed to solve the problem, and I saw the surgeon thinking that a surgeon's job does not include treating ordinary infections. I said that to him once. "A result of the surgery," he responded. "You're right," is what he meant, "but my professional ethics do not allow me to leave you to deal with this alone."

Suddenly he announced that as far as he was concerned I could go home. People could be lined up to care for me at home, and I could always call him if necessary. This made me a little nervous. Monday was discharge day. The same nurse told me once again that he thought it was too soon. I had just been given a drain, and he thought I ought to learn how to manage that first. That would take a couple of days. On Sunday the surgeon came by. He decided that now Tuesday would be a better day. During the Monday morning consultation, he said, "Everything looks good. You can go home tomorrow." The nurse and I exchanged surreptitious glances but neither of us said anything. Mar called to say that "today" was the day. She had to shift a lot of things around at work in order to pick me up from the hospital. It is assumed that home caregivers have nothing else planned.

So home we went. It felt cold outside after four weeks of an air-conditioned existence. Mar and I had talked about where to put the bed. We would use a sofa bed, with plenty of pillows. When we got home, I was so tired that I wanted to lie down right away. "How many pillows?" Mar asked, but I was already lying down. Immediately I felt a sharp stab in my back. I couldn't lie down, stood back up, lay down again, exhausted. Took some painkillers. That was better. We made the bed according to the right proportions and I tried to lie down again. No good. More painkillers. Tried to get through the night. It was difficult, but I was used to that.

"We've got to get a different bed," said Mar the next morning. But in order for that to happen, a consultant from the homecare service had to come over to evaluate the seriousness of the problems. The lack of sleep also led to other difficulties. "It can't go on like this," said Mar, and she called the surgeon. "He's not supposed to get worse just by being at home," she told him. I was readmitted to the hospital that afternoon. I felt relieved. The next day the surgeon was back at my bedside. "You look well," he reported. "It's the first time I've been able to sleep in two nights," was my response. The surgeon didn't know what else to do with me. He didn't say that, of course. After two days of nursing care, they sent me back home, where there was a state-of-the-art bed waiting for me: The head could be raised and lowered and the foot could, too, and there was even a hinge at the knees. Everything was operated by a single button. I was as pleased as Punch.

But soon a complication occurred. At night, I perspired heavily. I had to get into a fresh change of clothes three times a night. By the weekend, it was driving us around the bend, so we called our family doctor. The doctor who was standing in for him agreed to let us come over, and when he read my computer chart and looked at my body he fell silent. "I wouldn't touch this with a barge pole," I saw him thinking. "I'm referring you to the hospital emergency ward," he said. Ten minutes later, we were on familiar territory. The surgeon on duty was rather shocked when he saw what he saw. What problem did perspiration indicate if there was no fever? "Readmission," he suggested. That was too much for me. I suggested coming back the next day for an examination.

Everyday difficulties are nobody's problem. The specialists rarely see them, and if reports of them reach their ears, they let it be known that that's not what they're there for, or they insist on testing for something in their field. As for everything else, "that's why you have a family doctor." But a family doctor doesn't want to burn his fingers on someone with cancer, with tubes and bags hanging from his body. Then there's the homecare service. Home care is strictly regulated and scheduled. Ten minutes for a colostomy bag. "After one week you'll have to do it yourself." There are nurses who are specialized in colostomy bags, but they work in the hospital. They're just like the specialists. They teach you the basic principles, and after that the ward nurse has to take over. But they did it differently. "Wrong," said the specialists. "So I'll work it out for myself," I thought.

When it comes to day-to-day existence, the sick person is in no-man's-land. The boundary markers put up by the healthcare workers are far away. Just when the routine work on an illness is supposed to begin, the specialists withdraw. Back pain: No one seemed particularly concerned. So I had to engage a physiotherapist myself, and I listened to endless advice from others. Perspiration without a fever: That's the sick person's problem. And then there's the succession of other little things. When can I go outdoors, and how? At what temperature, and wearing what kind of clothing? The first time I went out I was back inside in two minutes, not shivering but rattling from the cold. I had no more control over my limbs, no fat to protect me. I was frozen to the bone. And that's what I seemed to consist of mostly. With a great deal of difficulty, I climbed into bed. After half an hour, my temperature was back to normal.

* * *

There is no health care for day-to-day problems. Specialists pass on the responsibility to family doctors, and family doctors to homecare workers. But homecare workers become specialists, too, so they also limit themselves to their own province. Sick people have to find their own replacements. Such replacements have already been invented by policymakers. They call them "informal" or "volunteer" caregivers. These caregivers may have a name, but they're not always available. And if they are available, they're not able to do everything. And there's still no name for the person who does all the chores in the day-to-day lives of the sick. Those chores end up on the shoulders of the partner and the sick person himself.

Sociologists know that "healthcare worker" refers to a spectrum that runs from top to bottom. This reference pattern is also part of our research—but within the borders of official health care. Many medical sociologists are medical conformists. We take as our area of research whatever is regarded as health care by the medical professionals.

That is why we don't realize that the reference pattern comes to an end at both extremes. The super-specialist doesn't know who might be able to carry on after he's done all he's able to do. The homecare worker doesn't know who might be able to carry on after he's done all he's allowed to do. The healthcare insurer speaks the language of "functions," but these functions are only arranged for, carried out, and paid for if they have names that sound medical. Anything without such a name remains uninsured, at least by the official caregivers.

Whatever is uninsured becomes work for the sick person and for the people around him. That work has been given names by Anselm Strauss and Juliet Corbin, who studied the day-to-day lives of the chronically ill: "illness management," the work involved in coping with the illness; "everyday work," making sure that life goes on as normal; and "making arrangements," delegating the work to others.

Sickness Skills

As its name suggests, health care is something that others do—mostly doctors and nurses, or so we think. Statutory regulations are also based on this assumption. The law on medical practitioners and a new law on professional practice in the healthcare services lay down rules for who can do what. The sick themselves are only mentioned passively. They are the ones who *get* the care. But a person who is ill knows how much he himself—uneducated, untrained, and unqualified—has to do.

In medical sociology, too, the sick have long been described as the receiving party. They are assigned the sick role, in society and by society.

They were the dependent ones who complied with the "professional dominance" of their principal caregivers, the doctors. When medical consultants were first subjected to interaction analysis, however, it was discovered that sick people actively play their own part, that they contribute the voice of their own environment, and that in so doing they sometimes interrupt the voices of the medical professionals.

But in this kind of analysis, the role of the sick was only studied in terms of their interaction with doctors, in their role as "patients." The "work" of the sick themselves became apparent only when they were examined on their own and not in direct contact with healthcare workers, when their everyday "managerial work" came out into the open. My own experience of illness has led me to believe that sociology should become even more every day and should deal with such things as the "skills" of the sick.

* * *

I had always looked with admiration at people who were able to roll from their wheelchair into a car. "Wrestling" was my word, but that didn't seem like the word they would choose. I thought about how difficult it would be for me as I watched them move into the car seat with such fluid grace. My admiration for that kind of dexterity was enormous.

I saw this because it took place in public, not hidden somewhere behind the scenes in the person's own house and sick room. Doctors apply all kinds of technology to the body without wondering whether the sick person can deal with what they have wrought. My doctor put several different tubes in my body, some with shut-off regulators, some with reservoirs with drain regulators attached, and some with import regulators and pressure injectors. There was an infection in my abdominal cavity so a drain had to be inserted, first in my buttock and later in my anus. My urination equipment didn't work, so a suprapubic catheter had to be installed with the outlet on my stomach. And another outlet was created for my colostomy bag. There were tubes hanging from all these outlets with bags to catch whatever came out of the tubes. But it didn't stay that way. First one tube was removed, then another. If my body refused to work as it was hoped, however, the tube would be reinserted. And sometimes with the addition of another tube.

Sometimes problems arose right away. On two occasions, two doctors and a nurse spent two hours inserting a drain leading to the infection in my abdominal cavity. The site of the infection was located with a scan, and the tube was ingeniously put into place and secured in my abdomen with barbs. "Secure" only applied to the operating table, however. Outside the operating room the barbs quickly slipped loose and the tube hung uselessly from my body. I felt it and knew it, sometimes within three minutes. But the doctors, in their extramural innocence, thought everything was secure.

Sometimes doctors only seem to be able to think about their patients when the patients are lying on a table or in bed. They don't seem to realize that once the operation is over, the patients have to keep on going, to get up and walk, even if it's only to the bathroom. Patients cannot allow themselves to stay in bed, certainly not after they're back home.

Staying in bed isn't such a problem in the hospital. I spent most of my first days in bed. The tubes and bags were all hanging from the bedside. The nurses did their work, emptying the bags according to a fixed schedule. The barbs and tubes stayed in place, almost of their own accord. But as soon as I became more mobile, I felt the barbs letting go and the tubes slowly sliding out of my body. Once it happened in a corridor of the hospital. Two hours of doctors' work, three minutes effective. The doctors had turned their attention to another recumbent patient by then. Maybe I can figure out how to deal with this, I thought. Once I pushed the tube back into my body. Once I managed to squirt some Betadine in via the loose tube in the hope that the iodine would make its way to the right place. It didn't, of course.

When I got home I had to take over the management of all my fluids. But how was I to get to the bathroom with three tubes and their three bags without losing them along the way? That required a great deal of concentration, as well as drawing up a plan of action before setting off. First move the one bag from the right side of the bed to the left, along with the tube. Then carefully stand up, making sure there's no strain on any of the tube connections. Then sit on the edge of the bed. Feel around to make sure all the hooks are unhooked. Carefully stand up next to the bed. Check once more to make sure I'm not stuck anywhere. Then, with one frame on the waistband of my pajama pants and the other frame in my hand, and the other hand supporting the colostomy bag, make my way to the bathroom step by step with three tubes connected to my body. Empty the bags one by one and then back to bed. The first time I attempted such an escapade I fell immediately into a deep sleep. The work had not yet become a skill. The great thing was that after a while a lot of this drudgery became routine. I didn't think about it anymore. I just did it, in flowing movements, and things rarely went wrong.

Then a doctor dropped in and said one of the tubes could come out. Euphoria. But soon I discovered that this reduction in tubes had disturbed my recently acquired routine. I found myself unexpectedly stuck in bed with a tube whose purpose I no longer seemed to remember. I kept searching on the lower right-hand side of my bed for something that was no longer there. After a few days, however, another routine was established, I was none the wiser, and everything went flawlessly.

Healthcare workers seem completely ignorant of such acrobatics. Of all my doctors, only my family doctor had seen me out of bed. The rest only saw me in bed. And not just the first ones: The surgeons who operated on me. The ward physicians, the doctors called in for consultations, the nurses who helped me get through the first days—all of them only knew me lying down. And the homecare workers who later came to tend to my wounds, to help me clean my equipment, and to teach me how to use it—they, too, usually saw me horizontal. But of all that maintenance work on my body, and especially the walking required to reach the place where that work could be done, the most difficult scenes from all those acts were the ones I did in isolation. Almost no one has ever seen that work. I have never heard anyone talk about it, and no one gave me any handy tips. It was work of my own invention.

It didn't stop with learning to deal with tubes and bags. Once I got home I had to come up with strategies for other things as well. For the pain in my back, for example. That, too, was something no one knew anything about. Painkillers, yes, but in a dosage that didn't help. So I took more, according to my own prescription. A woman friend recommended physiotherapy, which resulted in months of kneading for one hour's relief. Then there was the search for a way to lie in bed that was least painful, using pillows and plastic foam on a movable mattress to find a position I could tolerate, at least for a little while. Or sitting bolt upright in a chair, and searching for a chair that was suitable. The third one proved satisfactory. Finally I learned that only moving helped. First in bed, moving my buttocks up and down. And later out of bed. When I could walk again that proved the most effective. A wrecked body and a cane, thirty times up and down the hallway. Just like training.

When my urinary equipment refused to do its mechanized work after a while, I was faced with a different challenge. A catheter had already been inserted through my abdominal wall. Now the same plan was proposed, but I wasn't happy with it. After a great deal of whining on my part, a urologist suggested I do it myself by inserting a little tube into my urethra to enable me to pass water. Immediately enthusiastic. I practiced with a few nurses and it went well. Once at home, I stood in the bathroom every day and carried out a repertoire of precautionary measures before cautiously inserting a tube into my penis. But after a few days that, too, was readily accomplished. I was proud of my little tricks, although I could only talk about them and couldn't show them off. And even talking about them wasn't something I did often. Tricks with your dick, not a topic you easily launch into. And even when I did, it didn't impress people so much as horrify them, that such a thing was necessary.

* * *

To a great extent, health care is more self-care than healthcare workers, policymakers, and even sociologists like to admit. Sociologists write mainly about doctors, occasionally about pharmacists and nurses, and sometimes also about homecare workers, but by the latter they don't mean the sick themselves. In their writings, the sick are generally the recipients of care provided by others. When the sick are featured in the work of sociologists, it is mostly as people who respond to the care of others, only occasionally as people who react in some way, and rarely as people who take their care into their own hands—even though they are the ones who personally deal with a great many matters of health and illness, often at their own discretion. They have to solve many of these problems themselves. Illness is like traveling in unknown territory. Much of it is new, and travel guides are few and far between. The sick have a lot of sorting out to do, mostly by trial and error. That's not only because everyday sickness is an unexplored region. It's also because the work doesn't take place until the visitors have left. They don't share in the wisdom of the sick. They'd have to sort things out themselves if they were to become ill.

There are many health issues that people manage on their own—food and travel, for example. There's a lot of advice available, but many people refuse to take it. They have other priorities, or none. Even going to the doctor, the most important decision of all, is largely left to the sick themselves. The supposed medicalization of life and advancing preventive research have very little effect on this. The amount of work that people do themselves before going to the doctor is rarely the subject of the research. And if people do go to the doctor, then they themselves decide whether to follow the doctor's instructions or not. And a surprisingly, large number of people prove non-compliant in this regard:

They don't do what the doctor says, or they do it differently and take their medicines as *their* circumstances allow. And before you know it they're furiously working on ending their own lives.

Sociologists are making inroads into this world of the sick, but only gradually. And the world of self-care is even more difficult to penetrate. It was Strauss and Corbin who discovered the vast amount of work being done by the chronically ill. They broke this work down into types, each with its own phases: From "inventing" in the first stage to following "routines" in later, more stable phases. But very little has yet been done to identify sickness work and make it public. This will require a great deal more sociological research.

So everyday health care often involves self-care, sickness work. It's taken for granted that such work is unpaid, with a few exceptions. People in the Netherlands who provide their own health care are sometimes given a "personal budget." But that money is only meant to cover the costs of hiring care that is provided by others. Self-care is still charity.

Night Work

Medical sociology is a daytime sociology. I cannot remember ever having come across the word "night" in any of my literature. Most sociologists sleep at night, and society is closed for them then. But perhaps night is absent from their work because they think little happens there, they think other people sleep at night, too.

It isn't only medical sociologists who tend to overlook the night. The same is true of healthcare workers. They turn off the light in the sickroom and administer pills and shots to make sure light stays off. For a sick person in the hospital, the only help is the shadowy form of the "night nurse." They're there in case things go wrong at night. They know all about the nighttime tossing and turning of the sick, but the sick cannot actually call for them unless there's a serious problem. Sick people are forced to see nighttime as something to be gotten through. And that night of the sick is unexplored territory for medical sociologists.

* * *

Being ill upsets life's normal rhythms. It's no longer a matter of working during the day and sleeping at night. You don't work anymore. You sleep whenever sleep overtakes you, if you can fall asleep, and not if you can't fall asleep. I had my fixed times for sleep during the day:

At nine-thirty in the morning after a bath and breakfast, at one in the afternoon after lunch, and at seven-thirty in the evening after dinner. And often there were short naps in between, mostly after any kind of exertion and after treatment.

But nighttime was different. I never got any more than one or two hours of sleep. At first I tried everything. In the hospital I was first given sleep injections and later sleeping pills. But they didn't help. There were nights I thought I had been sleeping for quite a while, only to discover it had only been five minutes. So I quickly put together my own repertoire of pills. I began my preparations at eleven o'clock at night: One Seresta, half a sleeping pill, and two painkillers. I took them when all the din in the corridor had disappeared, when the night shift no longer came into ask how things had gone today. I tried to calm myself as much as possible, then in went the pills. They put me to sleep, usually until about twelve-thirty. If I got that far I was very happy.

But what to do after twelve-thirty? There wasn't much choice in the hospital. Usually there was someone lying next to me who almost always was a sound sleeper, which meant no TV. So I'd try to fantasize my way through the night. How delighted I was to hear rumbling in the corridor at 6 a.m., not so much because of the cup of tea that was on its way but because a day was breaking that would keep me busy. But sometimes I was alone. Then the light would go on, as well as the TV. I watched everything, as long as it was on the screen. It required little energy and it filled the time.

The same pattern occurred at home, except everything was a bit more protracted. I became a professional night worker. The eleven o'clock falling asleep ceremony was further developed. It was preceded by a period of meditation: Trying to achieve that sleepy feeling by thinking about nothing. Then a balanced number of whole and half pills. I became furious if anyone disturbed me in the middle of my ceremony. It took a lot of concentration and fussing to extract a single hour of sleep from the entire night.

After this brief sleep, the night hours arrived. Sometimes I got up and looked outside to see what kinds of folks wander around at night. At other times I started working, tinkering with my writings, hoping that would tire me out. Most of the time I just kept on going. Powerless, I turned to the radio and TV, the nocturnal refuge of the sick. With the help of the media I traveled through the night. This rhythm became more and more fixed: Five minutes of sleep and half an hour of TV, often until morning, when I switched to the radio and thereby fell asleep. The radio increasingly became my opiate. Listening to a talk show with my head on the pillow: that helped.

I owe a lot to nighttime TV. I watched everything, but everything wasn't much. Gradually I learned to find my way. First to Oprah. There was less and less of that as the almost unrestrained egotism finally hit home. Then CNN. Many repeats, so mostly things I had seen before and voices that set your teeth on edge. Then I discovered Belgium. I'm deeply grateful to the Belgians. At that time they were the only ones who repeated their evening news all night long. It was the time of Dutroux. My viewing habits became more and more a sociological study of Belgian judiciary practices. The rest of the Belgian news was also mainly about Belgium as well as its former African colony. There was more news about Africa than what we were seeing on Dutch TV. I'd watch their news broadcasts seven times in a row, and I slowly began to regard myself as an authority on Belgium. After a while, the things that had irritated me at first began to amuse me. "What are you going to do about it, Mr. Minister?" "Well, we're studying the case from every angle and we will not hesitate to take the necessary measures." "Thank you very much, Mr. Minister." Whenever this Minister of Justice was interviewed, I could predict every word of his response. When the same man was interviewed by a Dutch journalist, it immediately gave rise to a cultural conflict. The interviewer kept on asking questions, refusing to be put off. For a moment I was afraid the minister was going to attack him. But he controlled himself, this normally garrulous Belgian minister. The next day he was back among his own. And you could tell. I began to like the idea of researching cross-cultural interviews, comparing the Belgian approach with the Dutch. Something for later on.

And then there were sports. The supreme entertainment for sick fans. It's a distracting kind of excitement and it takes your mind off serious things. There's football, of course, but if you're sick you notice how little time it takes up. An hour and a half is soon over, and the recaps never last long. Tennis lasts longer, but when all is said and done it's just hitting a ball back and forth. For a while the Tour de France was my salvation. Uninterrupted reporting right from the start. It's was always a dream of mine to follow the Tour on wheels. Now I had the time, and there was no sense of guilt. For three weeks, I spent the day watching, alternating between Dutch and Belgian TV. In the evening, there were the recaps and at night the abbreviated version in the Belgian news.

In the end, it became more than entertainment. I felt unutterably happy. The Tour made me forget my worries about sleeplessness: If I couldn't sleep there was always Belgian TV and the Tour.

Mornings were difficult. At six o'clock the reruns stopped, and there was no fresh news on the radio until seven. Sunday was TV paradise. At eight o'clock, there was "Early Birds" and at ten a program about history. "I really should thank all those media people for pulling me out of the doldrums," I said to myself. But like so many resolutions I made when I was sick, nothing ever came of it.

* * *

Sick people have to find new ways to get by, and that includes making it through the night. If they succeed, their night is enriched. Illness is more than just affliction. The sick live in a different world than the healthy, and their nights are different, too. Sick people cross the borders of everyday life. Illness is like a vacation. You're on a journey, there's lots to see and to hear, you bring some of it back with you, and you find new people to love. And like being in another country, after a while you feel at home. It's almost as if you had gotten sick on purpose.

But there's plenty of everyday sickness work to do at night as well. Life must go on if sleep evades you. Disturbances have to be dealt with that are usually taken care of by others during the day. At night, a sick person is pretty much on his own. Because he has to do this work himself, he becomes an expert at "night work."

The procedures involved in night work deserve to be properly identified by sociologists, preferably by sociologists who are familiar with the night, such as those among them who are sick. These people are able to incorporate their own observations, as well as those of the sick people near them and the occasional nighttime healthcare worker, into their research. That work could make for excellent research material and could greatly benefit "every-night" health care.

CHAPTER 6

Control

Abstract More than half a century ago, Talcott Parsons coined the term "sickness role". One needs legitimation to be sick. The idea that one needs some kind of approval for being sick still exists. I had to do a lot of work as sick person. Activities that were trivial before I fell sick became difficult tasks. Slowly I learnt how to handle them, but I remained vulnerable. Sickness is not only a role, but also a trajectory that requires management and organization of yourself and others. In ordinary life, illness means uncertainty. What are you still able to do? You have to explore what your new borders are. After that, "normal" certainty returns.

Keywords Sickness role · Legitimation · Habituation · Uncertainty
Exploration

Necessary Redundancies

Some time ago, being ill was seen by medical sociologists as a "role," complete with a fully defined theory: that of the "sick role." Here the sick were given a number of rights as well as a number of duties. They might exhibit aberrant behavior, but they were expected not to do so deliberately and they were not held responsible for it. That was their first right. Their second right was that during their illness they were free to feel exempt from obligations. Illness was accepted as a legitimate reason for feeling so exempt. But then there were two duties. The first was that sick people

G. Nijhof, *Sickness Work*,
https://doi.org/10.1007/978-981-13-0326-5_6

must make an effort to get better. That implied—and this was the second duty—seeking competent help, from doctors, and agreeing to work with them. These rights and duties seemed to delineate the social world of the sick. But sociologists have started to think differently in recent years, compelled to do so by the sick people whose lives they investigated.

It was mainly the chronically ill who taught them that being ill is more a "trajectory" than a role—a trajectory, moreover, that runs through relatively unknown territory. This is because so many unexpected things happen when illness strikes, and because illness requires so much work, not only care and treatment but also organizational help, management. Usually the sick are not alone in doing this work. Being sick is mainly a collective undertaking. But the sick must also work on themselves. Sick people change. To be recognized as a sick person they have a lot of "biographical work" to do. To maintain their identity as a sick person they have a lot of legitimation work to do. As several books of medical sociology point out, sick people really have their hands full.

* * *

I experienced the pressure of illness and the work it requires in typical ways. I had to learn to live with my illness, not so much to process it as to cope with the uncertainties it evoked. All these uncertainties require work: paying attention to the faces of bystanders, asking questions, studying files, sounding out second opinions. A beginner in the world of the sick is assaulted by thoughts of doom. "Has it metastasized?" "Is there anything the doctors may have overlooked?" "Have they really told me everything?" I trained myself to handle these uncertainties by means of various tricks and dodges. What I also had to learn was how to unlearn—to break the habit of worrying, for example. That's easy to say in retrospect, now that I've become acquainted with the shape and features of my illness, now that I know what can happen, now that I've conquered my anxiety and hidden my worry beneath all the routines.

Serious ailments require both care and precautionary measures, taking steps to prevent things from happening. These can be considerable in the beginning, at least in the mind of the sick person. "Have I eaten enough salt and stocked up on enough fluids?" "What should I do if I suddenly feel sick?" "What if I realize I've forgotten to do something?" "Is there a chair I can sit on?" "Is there a bathroom with facilities?" "What if my colostomy bag loosens and the feces are released?" "Is there a change of clothes nearby?"

Because of these uncertainties, when I went back to work after a year of absence I brought all sorts of household items with me to the university: underwear and an extra pair of pants, a towel and a package of bandages, plastic bags and Q-tips, and reserve gear for my stoma (a baseplate to fasten to the skin, a pouch to be fastened to the baseplate, a clip to seal off the pouch, powder to staunch wounds)—everything I needed to make the mess invisible and odorless to others and manageable for myself. And then there was a supply of provisions associated with my condition: salted snacks, fluids, bouillon cubes in case of acute salt deficiency, an electric kettle to make the bouillon, a teapot, and a glass. Thus equipped, I arrived at my place of work. "Moving in?" I was asked by someone who didn't know of my situation.

That's how it went with so many of the things I undertook. My first visit to the theater was preceded by an exhaustive prelude. The best seat, I thought, was a corner seat. And was there an exit nearby if anything should happen to me? And would I be able to find it in the dark? And what if my colostomy bag gave way? And then something else: how could I prevent such a disaster? Eat earlier? Have a small evening meal at three in the afternoon to minimize my intestinal activity during the performance, now that my sphincter no longer worked? Or just eat after the theater? Or not at all? Precautionary measures weren't only for work and the theater. Every "new" venture—and that meant everything, after being hit by an ailment like this—had its own repertoire.

Much of this proved unnecessary later on. Nothing dramatic ever happened to me outside the house. So far all the stuff I dragged along with me was for naught. Almost none of the things I dreaded came to pass. Of course I do a great many preventive things that have now become routine, ordinary, as if I'd never done anything else. I eat and drink and live by different patterns. Once I did these things as precautionary measures; now I don't even remember how it was before.

Many of the measures I continued to be conscious of have proved unnecessary, at least not yet. And that "yet" is where my anxiety resides. A Dutch medical sociologist, Tjeerd Tijmstra (1987), came up with a nice term for this. People who undergo a medical procedure despite their hesitation, do it to avoid "anticipated decision regret." They're afraid that in the future they might be sorry for what they failed to do. This was true for me: taking precautionary measures to prevent me from regretting that I had not taken the measures in the first place. Trying to prevent the "if-only-I-had" feeling.

That is why I did so much unnecessary work, and why I still carry so many things with me. Of course the amount of baggage is constantly being reduced; I do this mainly when I'm about to embark on something I have never done before. I go to the movies just as I used to. I no longer waste my time worrying when I go out to eat. But when I have to spend two nights away from home, I still take everything with me. One night in a hotel seems like two weeks on tour. And vacations are practically emigrations.

I had just recovered from another minor operation and I was about to go away on vacation. I had misgivings, but Mar really wanted to go and I really wanted her to get what she wanted. She had spent two years being ill with me, which meant no vacation at all. We booked a vacation in Greece near a woman friend, who lived close by and was married to a Greek. If emergency struck, she would know how to navigate the Greek healthcare system. And because she worked for a travel agency, she would be able to arrange for a return flight if things got out of hand. But what else should we be thinking about? Would the baseplate on my colostomy bag loosen if the temperature went above a hundred? Would my skin become inflamed? I called the supplier of my "equipment." He, too, thought the temperatures in Greece were excessively high. But he had a "skin prep" that can form an intermediate layer between baseplate and skin to prevent complications. Had I thought of taking backup equipment with me? In case the suitcase and I ended up in two different places and I had to spend days without it? A whole truckload of salted food was coming with me. The Greeks can't be trusted as far as salt is concerned, or so I thought. Maybe a little more salty cheese? And a piece of salted ham? They're sure to have bottled water, right? And don't plan on being too active in the hot Greek weather. I had already told Mar that I'd probably have to stay on our balcony in the shade, reading and looking out at the sea. These were the kinds of precautionary measures I envisioned.

And so my preparations progressed, with images of calamities and the appropriate measures to avoid them. I didn't even purchase a new travel guide. As long as all went well with my ailment I'd deal with the rest when it happened.

I have rarely done so much in so short a time as I did on that vacation. It began with two walks up the mountains in the heat of the day. We packed some salted snacks and drinks in a bag and decided to give it a try. And it went fine. Then we rented a car. First we visited the friend in Lefkas. And as usually happens when visitors from home arrive, we spent the whole day being shown the sites, including her husband's remote native village. Got through the whole day completely unprepared. Drove back to our hotel much too late over a dark and winding road and arrived at midnight. Much to my surprise everything went well. Then we went into the interior by car. There were excavations to see and villages that a guide had recommended to us. A whole day of heavy driving and walking, getting back late once again by means of an unlit mountain road. And because that went so well, we signed up for a two-day excursion to the Meteora monasteries. The thought still occurred to me: "What if something goes wrong in the bus, or if I suddenly have to empty my bag?" I told the guide I had "health problems" that necessitated leaving the bus abruptly. But before I could finish talking, she interrupted me with a face that said, "What are you worried about?" "Our driver can find a place within two minutes where you can take care of things," she confided. "Children are always having to go to the bathroom unexpectedly." And "of course" the hotel room in the interior came complete with bathroom. What else could happen to me? I couldn't think of a thing. And nothing happened.

Ailments like mine are "unnecessary work" ailments. Precautionary measures are almost always redundant. A lot of work for nothing. But not entirely. They do provide peace of mind, which is why the measures were not redundant. Conditions like mine are "necessary redundancy" ailments. In order to move about freely and without agitation, a certain amount of work has to be done that afterwards seems needless. To make sure nothing ever does happen, a great deal of foresight is required.

But I find that the longer I live with my condition, the less attention I pay to that foresight. I do think about what could happen, but I don't often go into detail. I do imagine various situations, but rarely with the accompanying images of filth and stench. Apparently that's going too far. I wave that aside. I've consulted with myself about what I should to do if anything were to happen to my colostomy bag in a public place. Should I run away and ignore everyone? Should I leave the mess behind with the owner of the establishment and travel homewards without letting him know? Should I inform the theater personnel of the excrement lying on their floor? Should I leave my fellow theatergoers to fend for themselves? Should I myself ask for a cloth? Should I ever show my face in that place again? What happens after I've left? Should my companion try to explain what happened? Or would Mar rush out of the building with me? Will the owner of the place apologize to the guests for the inconvenience? What will people think after I'm gone? I'm asking all these questions now in such detail because now I'm typing and reflecting on them. Back then I thought about them all every day. But even then I quickly zapped to something different, as you do when you're watching a TV show you'd rather not see. My precautionary consciousness has apparently become almost unconscious. I leave my nightmares out of my scenarios. Precautionary measures must not be allowed to go too far, which is why I've become daring once again. Now I do things without thinking about them, things I would have regarded as foolhardy awhile back. The precaution is under control. I have now set a boundary around my worry. What lies behind it has been rendered practically unthinkable.

* * *

The purpose of precaution is to allow you to dare, and the purpose of daring is to learn that precaution is redundant, to dare to do something without taking precautions. Sick people have to learn to take things for granted again. Being chronically ill means unlearning the tendency to be too cautious. Sickness work involves breaking free of redundancies. Being ill is learning to dare. It makes sick people brave. But bravery in turn makes sick people more aware of their vulnerability. They're afraid that by shouting down their cautiousness they will actually diminish it. And sooner or later, they fear, those precautionary measures are going to be necessary after all.

Illness makes the vulnerability of everyday existence more palpable. Illness interferes with the way we take everyday existence for granted. After a while we do begin taking it for granted again, to a certain extent. But the vulnerability is always lurking. Illness breeds vulnerability.

Hiding and Habituation

Illness does not leave the body untouched. Where the body was once unblemished there are now scars. Where there once were flowing forms there are now pieces missing, or pieces added on. This is the bizarre body that sick people have to go on living with. Fortunately ours is a culture in which much of the body is normally concealed. But clothing is capable of covering only some of this disorder.

Medical sociologists pay remarkably little attention to such physical disorder. The best research has been done by a sociologist who did more than medical sociology alone, Erving Goffman (1963). He showed how inventive people have been in dealing with facial deformities. They have to. They're being seen.

Partners are accustomed to seeing more of the bodies of their injured partners than others are. For them, concealing the body is unusual. So they are the ones on whom bodily injury has the most impact. They see what is being hidden.

Something must be done about this. New forms of concealment are being developed. Concealment happens physically, but mostly it happens symbolically. The process of "habituation" renders scars invisible and deformations normal—normally.

* * *

My body didn't get any better looking after my operations either. At first my belly was a regular oil field: drills, indentations, and excavations, and a plumbing system on top of it all. My body had also become quite thin, no more than skin and bones. In my conversations with Mar I spoke about "the" body. She kept reminding me that the body was mine. Apparently that was something I didn't want to acknowledge.

You can get used to just a physical injury. What was troubling was the body's appearance. I had lost fifteen kilos in a short time, and I hadn't had much surplus to start with. My head felt like a skull, my arms hung down like slats, my shoulders stuck through my skin, my rib cage could be seen in full detail, my buttocks were like loose sacks, and my legs were stilts. My thighs were gone completely. The ratio of skeleton to flesh was high. I just didn't want to look at it anymore. Fortunately I didn't often have to. Mirrors are not widespread among the sick. Feeling my body was quite enough. And I only did that when there was no getting around it.

I was shocked the first time I was forced to look at myself, standing in the bathroom in front of the mirror. "So thin!" But immediately another thought came to mind. "As long as the cancer treatment is going well." And the daily concerns distracted me, too. The body had to be cared for and quickly covered with a sheet. Almost no one saw it, only the passing nurses, and they seemed accustomed to such things. They hardly knew any better. For others it was the body under the sheet, except for the head.

The first public confrontation with the body came when my colostomy nurse found it necessary to "let the partner have a look at the stoma." After all, she would have to live with it, too. That struck me as a psychohygienic idea. So we made an appointment. "Let's do it in the bathroom," said the nurse. The toilet was there as well. I knew that, but I had momentarily forgotten it. So there we sat, the three of us, each one on a stool. Two women fully clothed and me without clothing, under the neon lighting, naked, not only because I wasn't wearing clothes but mainly because my colostomy bag had been removed. There we sat, like stones. Me bare, cold, thin, with a little red lump of flesh on my belly where excrement could come out at any moment. Contrary to her usual practice Mar didn't ask any questions. Right to the end, she didn't say a thing. And all the nurse did was provide an explanation. I no longer remember anything of what she said, and Mar doesn't either. When the nurse decided the session was over, she left the bathroom. So did Mar. I got dressed and made my way back to bed. I saw the nurse engaged in a lively conversation with my roommate's visitor. Apparently she knew him. I collapsed into bed, completely worn out. The nurse stopped by to say a few friendly words to me. Still bewildered, I told her that perhaps Mar would get used to it. "She's a psychotherapist," I added. "Angry too late—again," I thought hours later.

But all was soon forgotten. We had other things on our minds: organizing daily life, the everyday hassle of dealing with my body. The first thing was to get back on my feet and try to make myself a little presentable. I don't believe I had even thought of *that* yet. In the beginning it's more working than thinking. The body's unsightliness is a minor concern when it's in need of care.

Once I got home I preferred to keep my colostomy bag hidden. Gradually Mar got a look at it every now and then. I had begun to follow a strategy without ever planning to do so. At first I got dressed with my back to her. If my colostomy bag required attention, I went into the bathroom and closed the door behind me. After a while Mar walked in on me occasionally. At first I shouted that I was "busy." Later I stopped doing that, but I did stand with my back to her. Sometimes I walked around with the bag on my stoma without even thinking about it, but only when the colostomy bag had just been emptied, not when it was visibly full. Life with a damaged body is something that has to be reinvented. And once it's been reinvented, it has to become normal.

But life goes on, as it always does. I've almost forgotten what it used to be like. I no longer remember it having been all that different. Apparently, a human being is a master at becoming acclimated to unusual things and treating them as normal. They've even become more normal than I initially felt possible. In the hospital bathroom I thought my colostomy would mark me, but now it has shrunk in significance. It's like living in my new house: I don't find myself smiling all the time anymore, and likewise I'm not constantly moping about what's wrong with my body. Almost everything became ordinary, as if it had never been otherwise. This is the way calamities are covered over. That ability to settle in and get used to things is really a blessing.

* * *

Sociologists often claim to reveal things that are hidden: articulating concealed intentions, demonstrating the pretense of civilization, unveiling backstage conduct, disclosing secretive behavior.

As far as I can tell, we medical sociologists have only been partially successful in this regard. We know how doctors leave the body in tatters, but we only rarely discuss what that means for the people involved or how they deal with the situation. We know that people masking their illnesses, but exactly how they do it is seldom investigated. Ever since Goffman we have known something about how people handle deformities, but very little research has been done on the reactions to deformities beneath the clothing. How people cope with deformities caused by illness and treatment, how they hide them and avoid them, how they exaggerate and minimize them in their heads, how they are embarrassed by them or make fun of them, how the deformities are concealed yet are visible anyway—all this has yet to be spelled out.

If concealing deformities is difficult or is no longer possible, other techniques must be devised. And if these techniques don't help, there's still something else to try: habituation. With habituation, deviation becomes normal, at least for the deformed. But there are more people involved in this process than the deformed person alone. For all of them there is plenty of work to be done in the search for the precarious balance between maximizing and minimizing, between exposing and concealing, between being observed and carrying on unobserved.

Exploring Borders

If someone is diagnosed with an illness according to medical criteria, then doctors regard that person as ill. In that case one thing is certain: treatment. But in ordinary life things are different. In ordinary life an illness often means uncertainty. What are you still able to do? Are there things you should stop doing? Will you still be able to do things tomorrow that you were able to do today? Can you make plans for two weeks from now? To be ill is to be uncertain. If a sick person isn't uncertain yet, he will be soon. There's no avoiding it. And the people around him will be uncertain, too.

Sociologists have searched for the causes of these uncertainties. They have found several: the unpredictability of the course of the illness, lack of insight into the possible ways of coping with the illness (Robinson 1988: 74–85; Calnan 1984) the unpredictability of the reactions of others, the disruption of one's personal biography (Bury 1982), and the uncertainty of healthcare workers. The uncertainty harbored by the sick with regard to the possibilities and prospects lying before them is given much less attention.

* * *

What am I still able to do? What will I be able to do in the future? What will I never be able to do again? With my particular illness, the borders that once were clear became blurred. After my operation I could do practically nothing myself. I was helped at every turn. "Do you think you might be able to wash yourself in bed?" one of the nurses asked me after about four days. I had never even thought I'd be able to wash myself again. It went better than expected. I felt like a whole person once more, lying there in that bed. It was a feeling that was quickly snatched out from under me. Time to get out of bed. After one meter I was right back in, exhausted. The next day I slowly went a bit farther. After a week and a half I went out to the corridor alone. "My, my, Mr. Nijhof, you're doing very well!" I had expected a round of applause. After two meters in the corridor I staggered back. Two days later I shuffled even farther, with Mar. In a month I was walking relatively normally. Up and down the corridor with a walking stick, and the wall within reach, felt normal enough to me. I left the hospital and went outside, a walking stick in one hand and Mar's arm in the other. I couldn't walk alone yet, and I couldn't imagine daring to go any farther than within sight of our house. The first paces outdoors were baby steps. How could I get so tired from doing so little? And be so cold from going out alone? But under pressure from Mar I did go out for a real walk. Once I got out, I wanted to go farther and farther. Too far, as it turned out. I had to be picked up by car and driven home.

Then came the first car rides. Mar behind the wheel, me beside her, seated on a contoured cushion and armed with several other appliances. Suitable food and drink in the back seat. Seeing real foliage for the first time. Back home after an hour, exhausted. Went to bed immediately and slept for hours.

Only then did the thinking begin. Would I ever be able to bike again? Would the desire for sex ever return? Would I ever be able to go out with my colostomy bag? And on vacation? Camping seemed out of the question, but hotels? Would I be able to go back to work in Amsterdam with this diverted intestinal network? What would I do in a crowded train if my colostomy bag were suddenly to fill up? Could I give university lectures again with such a demanding body?

Everything improved, but very slowly. The most minor complications set me back weeks. For a long time there was no progress at all. I spent months in pain and misery. But after those months Mar talked me into spending two days away, including an overnight stay. We had to bring all sorts of things with us. I had taken every complication into account. But it all went better than expected. We walked for half an hour. There were no complications. And cafes are good places for resting, too.

These border crossings always took place during vacations. After almost two years we went abroad for the first time. There the walks were much longer than I anticipated. I wanted to go over that hill, to Lychos. So off we went. Wrestled my way to the top, resting on stones every fifty meters. It was no more difficult for me than it was for Mar. And it got better and better. The return trip was too much for me. Came back by boat. Almost every problem was immediately solved, against all my expectations. Two days later and I set my sights on that fort, high up on the other mountain. At first it seemed impossible, but I reached it easily. A glorious feeling. Not because I could do it, but because I now knew that the borders I had insisted on drawing in my mind could now be crossed. Life was open again, not screened off by imaginary borders of I-can't-do-it, or I-don't-know-if-it's-possible, or I-don't-think-so. No more resisting what Mar-hopes-I-can-do.

When the fort proved within reach, I thought maybe that nature reserve several kilometers away would be feasible. Set out alone. This time, however, I *had* reached too far. I tired out sooner than I had expected. I was tired longer, too. Maybe I had had too little to drink? Or too little salt? I sat a lot, ate some more, took another drink, but nothing helped. Had I done too much yesterday? Did I need company? Should I curb my ambitions?

After two days at home I came down with the flu. I'd never in my life been bothered by the flu, and this was my third bout in a short time.

Completely out of shape, I thought. Back pain again. Shaky legs. After ten days I finally went outside for the first time with Mar. Felt like an old man, and looked like one, too. Had it been too much? Had I overtaxed my body? Or was this just a worse kind of flu?

One week later, however, we took a bike trip to Heusden, a small fortified town in the south of the Netherlands, as we had planned earlier. It was a long ride, and I wasn't a bit tired. Biked farther than I had in years. The borders suddenly seemed to have shifted. But for how long?

* * *

To be ill seems like a return to childhood. The borders are still unknown, and it's all a matter of trial and error. You want to go farther than your ability allows, or even farther than you dare. You lose your way, get lost, stay inside for a little while, and then go out again to explore the borders again, and what is quite normal today was what you didn't dare to do yesterday. To be ill is to be constantly re-framing a new world. Old borders no longer apply, new ones have yet to be drawn. To be ill is to try things, to "explore borders." Fear makes you hesitant, courage makes you reckless, injury makes you wiser, just doing something makes life normal again.

Sociologically, long-term illness is the domain of the unregulated, of the non-institutionalized. Life is no longer the life that people were accustomed to living. Life has to be rediscovered. People with a long-term condition do not enter a programmed existence. They can't count on having everything done for them. Not only do they themselves have to figure a great many things out, find out what works for them, but their friends and relations do, too. They have to learn what they can expect, what they can demand, and what they'll have to give up. Learning these things is tedious, because the illness—and therefore living with the illness—is always changing. Anyone who lives with a sick person has to be ready to welcome limitations—and uncertainty as well.

In my research on people with Parkinson's disease I had already noticed that in their life stories they spoke often and emphatically of the "ordinariness" and "naturalness" of life before they became ill (Nijhof 1995). Back then they did "what everybody else did," they said, "spontaneously" and "without even thinking about it." But with Parkinson's that naturalness was constantly being eroded. The comfort of the ordinary had disappeared. The world outside the home in particular, which they had once taken for granted, had become untrustworthy for people with Parkinson's. Going outside the home became a burden because of the constant need to beware and think ahead. The simplest outing became a major event that required so much planning that it turned into an expedition, at least for a short time. Because the outside world was untrustworthy, it became for them what nighttime in the city is for women. Just as women—and increasingly more men—plan their nighttime route through the city, choosing well-lit streets and avoiding suspicious areas, so people with Parkinson's go over their proposed route beforehand and ask themselves whether the streets aren't too wide for their stiff and unpredictable bodies to cross, or whether the sidewalks aren't too high for their rigid legs to step onto. What had been a natural world was now a place of deliberation for people with this illness. They had to carefully consider all their comings and goings in the world. The trustworthy world had become a world of uncertainty.

The flip side of those uncertainties are the problems of legitimation. A person's borders may be uncertain but they must constantly be negotiated. What is it that he cannot ask of other people? What can he legitimately give up? What can he legitimately ask others to do for him? This requires constant work, mainly the work of explaining and justifying. Long-term illness seems like a long period of unlegitimized uncertainty. But after exploring the borders with others, and tacitly negotiating with them, the sick person will find that much of the normal certainty returns.

References

Bury, M. 1982. Chronic Illness as Biographical Disruption. *Sociology of Health & Illness* 4: 167–182.

Calnan, M. 1984. Clinical Uncertainty: Is It a Problem in the Doctor–Patient Relationship? *Sociology of Health & Illness* 6: 74–85.

Goffman, E. 1963. *Stigma, Notes on the Management of Spoiled Identity.* Englewood Cliffs: Prentice-Hall.

Nijhof, G. 1995. Parkinson's Disease as a Problem of Shame in Public Appearance. *Sociology of Health & Illness* 17 (2): 193–205.

Robinson, I. 1988. *Multiple Sclerosis.* London: Tavistock.

Tijmstra, T. 1987. Het imperatieve karakter van medische technologie en de betekenis van de geanticipeerde beslissingsspijt [The Imperative Character of Medical Technology and the Meaning of Anticipated Decision Regret]. *Nederlands Tijdschrift voor Geneeskunde* 131: 1128–1131.

CHAPTER 7

The Outside World

Abstract The hospital is not a place of medicine and health care alone. It is filled with people of flesh and blood. You can hear crying as well as laughter. There can be noise, both day and night. Meetings take place, with nurses and other personnel, with other patients and with visitors, sometimes pleasant, sometimes disturbing. It all affects your mood and well-being. Your visitors ask how you are. What to answer? Often it is best to pretend optimism; you don't want to embarrass or burden them with your pain and insecurity. Anyway, words are always a problem. When things go really badly it is best to keep silent. Sociologists, however, focus mostly on spoken words; they should listen more to the silence.

Keywords Hospital · Nurses · Doctors · Visitors · Laughter
Optimism · Noise · Silence

Gravity and Levity in the Hospital

Hospitals strike us as institutions where everything is focused on health care. The people who work there seem to do nothing but caring for the sick, and the people who occupy beds there seem to spend the whole day being sick and being patients. Is that because the hospital is easiest to organize along unidimensional lines? Because only the health care is designed organizationally? Because it would be more difficult if patients

G. Nijhof, *Sickness Work*,
https://doi.org/10.1007/978-981-13-0326-5_7

also had private lives: if they didn't only lie in rooms but lived on their own, with the freedom to withdraw if they wanted and to keep their own schedules ("not available for care today")?

Nursing homes are already wrestling with this problem. Casually walk into a resident's room? Serve residents only coffee, and not beer if they ask for it? Didi van Nee, a student of mine, encountered this demarcation problem when she observed the caregivers in such a nursing home. Many of their staff discussions had to do with what could and could not be asked of them, what was and was not part of their job description. Their work is not yet so professionalized that everyone—they themselves or those in their care—unquestionably accepts what their work comprises, as is the case with doctors. The borders of their work must be constantly reassessed. And because the residents of the nursing homes don't know where the borders lie either, conflicts are constantly arising that must be negotiated over and over again.

The hospital's organization seems more unvarying: medicine and health care, and nothing else. That's what most sociologists think as well. They study hospitals almost exclusively in terms of institutions for the sick. They're mainly interested in the professional conduct of doctors, and what patients think of it. But some sociologists have seen more. The Dutch sociologist Lammers spoke of a "caste society." Renée Fox (1959) called attention to the "humor" of surgeons in the operating room. Glaser and Strauss (1965) found that awareness of their patients' approaching end caused healthcare workers to distance themselves from them. Sudnow (1967: 61–116) discovered the "social death" that manifested itself in dealing with the dying. And Berg (1992) showed that what at first glance seems like treatment decreed by medical science is in reality behavior that is regulated by trivialities. The hospital is not involved in medicine and health care alone.

Medical knowledge and health care are put on display for all to see, however, while the private is carefully screened off. This is also evident on a smaller scale, when healthcare workers in the hospital act with "gravity" while letting their "levity" show behind the scenes.

* * *

A hospital is a serious place at first glance. People hear devastating news there. And things happen there that are usually only seen on the battlefield, like people dying. In the hospital, however, most of this takes place behind closed doors.

Nevertheless, you do see people walking through the corridors crying. Others look as if they were about to burst into tears. Some show signs of panic. I got lost when I first heard I had cancer. But you also see people who seem oblivious to any serious problems, whose faces suggest that misfortune had never touched them. There are those who seem to be lying there for the sole purpose of meeting up with old friends. And those who apparently have grown closer to their neighbors. There are also those who look as if they haven't spoken to each other in a long time. And those who are visibly concerned about the fate of others. And moving around among them are doctors, nurses, physiotherapists, dieticians, X-Ray technicians, and whatnot, all being serious and professional.

But every now and then you can still hear merry laughter in the hospital, including from the people working there. Healthcare workers are people, too. They have an ordinary working day, and they try to get through it pleasantly, just like any other employee.

Laughter isn't a problem as long as the sick and the caregivers are both involved. It means the problems are not very acute. The tension is momentarily broken. But if the laughter is one-sided the situation quickly becomes awkward. Two worlds collide. The laughter of the laughing person makes the serious person look ridiculous. Conversely, to be serious in the face of laughter is to treat the laughing person with contempt. Laughing people repudiate the person who is serious, and vice versa. Serious people shut out those who laugh, and laughing people shut out the serious. When one of these worlds forces its way into the other, tension arises.

Cheerfulness is different than laughter. Cheerfulness has the color of hope, as with the nurses who enter the sick room with a lighthearted "good morning." This is lightheartedness whose only limit is that of approaching death. Most patients are cheered up by it.

The person who does the laughing is also a factor. The cleaning ladies seem the least encumbered. They're not expected to know a great deal about the people whose rooms they are cleaning. I never heard a single cleaning lady come into my room and ask me how I was doing. One of them once remarked, "So, back again?" when I was re-admitted three days after having been discharged. But that was the only time. They have their fun among themselves, without including the sick. They seem to have come from another world. They're outsiders. They don't have to comply with the hospital rules. They laugh whenever they want. They're not healthcare workers.

It's mainly doctors and nurses who belong to the world of the sick. The sick are there for them alone, and they are there exclusively for the sick, or so it seems. They constitute a closed hospital world in which each plays his own role and each limits himself to his own domain. The borders are seldom crossed. Even when they are, the trespassers always stay close to home: "Do you work in health care, too?" a surgeon once asked my wife. One of my nurses did come to talk to us once, but always when work was over and only on Sundays, when there was less to do, and with barely a glimpse at her watch. "Not much to do" and "unseen" were apparently her borders.

But the division of worlds doesn't apply all the time or everywhere. The hospital is a workplace, but it's also a place for coffee and tea, for taking breaks, for coming and going, for vacation (and especially for coming back from vacation), for chatting about one's own life, about the happy and the serious things, about children who are born and experiences with the older ones, but also about everyday sorrows, loves that failed, cars that won't run.

A sick person who is uncertain about his future is well advised to stay clear of anyone with the urge to talk loudly and at length about his vacation, at least that's my opinion. The contrast is too great. But a person in pain also tends to shield himself from the laughter of others. Laughter comes across as thoughtlessness, to him and to those lying near him. Someone who is in pain, or who sees someone else in pain, can get very angry about the "limitless" pleasure of others.

The hospital has found a way to deal with this. Usually the worlds of gravity and levity are kept separate. People who are dying are given a private room. People who have just been operated on can be spotted in the corridor from far away: a bed with tubes and bottles, surrounded by serious-looking attendants. And usually you can tell from their faces that levity is out of place here, so passers-by know how to behave.

But sometimes things go wrong. My operation was on a Tuesday. Because there was hemorrhaging the operation was put on hold. And so was I. I was kept sedated for the whole night in a recovery room. But apparently the anesthesia wasn't so strong that everything escaped me. I heard people walking around. I heard machines, not only mine but also other people's. I heard doors banging. I heard people fiddling with some kind of device. I also heard a doctor make a phone call, and sometimes I caught snatches of his conversation, and of his laughter.

This is how I'm writing it down now, but that night I had different thoughts. I thought the banging door was the door leading outside. I heard people walking outside on the gravel. And once I heard someone squeeze a machine through the door with a great deal of difficulty. Suddenly I knew. The people coming in were nurses who had begun their shift. One of them had a motorbike that had broken down. And because there wasn't much to do at night, he started fiddling with his motorbike, or so I thought. Apparently he couldn't get it to work because he kept on fiddling with it. Other people kept talking to the fiddling nurse. "They're giving him advice," I thought.

I was overcome with rage. There I was, stricken with a fatal disease, and the best that the staff could do was to work on a motorbike. Once that idea hit me I knew I'd never get a wink of sleep, or so I thought. Once I thought what I had thought, there was no stopping me. The rage swelled. Next to me I thought I heard a woman groaning. "Why don't they help her, for heaven's sake? What a bunch of jerks." The doctor kept coming up to my bed. He'd say something like, "How are you doing, Mr. Nijhof?" Getting angrier by the minute, I said to myself, "The next time I hear 'Mr. Nijhof' I'm going to give him a piece of my mind." And I did: "There are people here who are critically ill and they're being treated disgracefully." And I added, "The nurse is working on a motorbike, for crying out loud." I also let him know that I wasn't happy about the way the groaning woman next to me was being treated. "A motorbike?" he asked. The doctor listened to me and didn't say a word. Apparently he was used to night owls, and that did little to improve my mood.

Then the next working day started, the operation was resumed, and for a long time I was aware of nothing. A few days later and back on my ward, a nurse told me she heard that I had had a difficult time in the recovery room. The doctor she spoke with had told her that I had complained about the noise. "You were right," she said. "It's very noisy there. People stomp around all over the place," and "they work with a lot of machines in there," and "sometimes, when things are really bad, people there are up all night." Calm explanation. Nobody blamed. It seemed the recovery room doctor had not responded to my "disgraceful" with his own "disgraceful." Apparently there was sympathy for a patient who complained about the threshold between two worlds being crossed, even if one of those worlds was invented.

Not everyone was so sympathetic. A few days after my operation a dietician came by to tell me I had to follow a diet because of my colostomy: 1300 grams of salt a day and 2.5 liters of fluid. She explained this in terms of sandwiches—salted raw ham was best—and in terms of cups and glasses and the number of cc's they held, and the difference between mugs, also in terms of cc. I was still drowsy from the morphine, and I had a visitor at the time who was listening in. The dietician's implacable tone annoyed me, as did the time she had chosen to see me. Couldn't she have come at a quieter moment? She asked me if I now knew what I was to eat and how much. "Let's start with breakfast," she said. "What do you put on your bread?" "Jam," I said, irritated and unthinking. She blanched. Had she given me her entire lecture for this? I tried to concentrate and answer the rest of her questions to her satisfaction. Now she had to leave, she said, "on vacation to the Canary Islands." She didn't expect "to meet me there," but she hoped I'd have "a good time," too. She had crossed the border between gravity and levity. Flabbergasted, I said nothing in return.

But it was visitors who crossed the border the most. Many of them were just plain scum. Not on purpose, I think, but scum out of awkwardness and carelessness and whatever causes it. Among the visitors were a couple who sat at the bedside of my roommate, fresh from the operating table, and droned on for an hour about their new car. My roommate had an ailment that would prevent him from ever being able to drive a car again. He could barely even walk, but he gave me a colorful description of doing his gardening while dragging himself around on his backside. How did such an extremely engaging man end up with acquaintances like these? And then there was the couple who talked for an hour about their successful child. "How good you look," they said to my neighbor upon their arrival. But that was the end of it. For the rest of the visit they talked about themselves and their child. Visitors like these deny the world of gravity as if it didn't exist, and consequently as if the person they're visiting doesn't exist. Usually the sick don't have much to say in return.

Sometimes I tried to take a bit of distance from my anger. "What a great subject this would make for a lecture on medical sociology," I would say to myself. Science as a suppressor of emotion. But how much better it would be if I were to use that sociology to discover how the worlds of gravity and levity, of sickness and health, of the lives of the patient and the public, of sorrow and callousness, are usually kept apart in hospitals.

* * *

How are the borders managed in hospitals by the people who frequent them? The border of seriousness and worry? The border of fun? How do they separate the public from the private? Where are people seen strictly as sick patients, and are therefore treated as such, and where can they be personal, be themselves? Do they only speak privately with their visitors, or are they sometimes private with their caregivers as well? And their caregivers with them? And if so, under what circumstances? Where can the caregivers be personal? Under what circumstances can they make jokes and laugh?

This is not a problem for hospitals alone. Every organization has—in Goffman's (1959) terms—its "frontstage" and its "backstage." The organization exists to serve official purposes, but people can't be official all the time. The organization organizes official things, but it also officially organizes informal things. This is why there are coffee breaks as well as cafeterias, corridors, collective bathrooms, and chatting areas such as secretarial rooms. But sometimes people organize private places on their own, places where they can enjoy themselves. They may need to get away for a while, mentally or physically. They organize places for diversion, for clandestine dealings. They visit with people who are easy talkers. They create their own "underlife."

Pointing this out isn't nearly as difficult as trying to figure out how it happens: local, time-specific, and differing from institution to institution—the kind of hospital research that's perfect for sick sociologists.

Private conversations with healthcare workers can only take place at the patient's bedside. But doctors almost never carry on such conversations there. Nurses are somewhat more amenable. They often distinguish the private from the public in their work, in my experience. Nurses will sometimes tell you something private while they're doing something with your bed, or caring for you in some way (it would have to be routine work, though), or in an effort to distract you from the pain involved in their treatment. In that case, however, the private talk becomes professional again. Because doctors in hospitals don't do routine work, or at least they don't seem to, they are less likely to speak privately. And if they do, it's not *their* private life they talk about but the private lives of their patients.

The private lives of healthcare workers take place out of sight of the patients, but not always out of earshot. Chattering and laughter about ordinary funny things come in from the corridor, from around the corner, usually from their own rooms. That's where you hear the tension-breaking laughter that would otherwise be deemed inappropriate in the rooms of patients.

The Optimism of Illness

We have a special relationship with illness. Illness is dreadful and we want it to be over and done with. So we propagate hope, and we do all we can to keep that hope alive. But we are also afraid of illness, and we prefer not to think too much about it, certainly not in too much detail. We'd rather not be confronted with it, or talk about it. If we absolutely have to, we speak in terms of "progress," and—if there is no progress—of "hope" and "optimism."

Research has shown that this optimism and hope is mainly to be found among doctors, nurses, and the sick themselves. The Dutch sociologist Abram De Swaan (1990: 31–56) was first to confirm this in his hospital study with his "regime of hope," followed by Anne-Mei The (2002) in her study of the hospital treatment of people with lung cancer. But hope and optimism on the part of bystanders is rarely discussed in the existing research, perhaps because researchers seldom include them, and when they do, it's in terms of the "support" they are believed to provide.

* * *

In the beginning I didn't have much to tell my acquaintances about how I was doing. But the faintest indication of "well" proved to be enough of an answer. Some people knew beforehand that things were going well. "I spoke with A and heard you were doing well. Thank goodness." People like that are almost impervious to contradiction. But I knew these would have been my own words if I had been on the other end of the phone. Being ill is a play for two actors, both of them dedicated to fending off suffering.

After a while I still wasn't sure how I should respond. Usually I began with a hopeful report. "It's going better." I thought that was better than "well." Optimistic, yet restrained. But sometimes even that was too much of a good thing. Then for a while it was "reasonably well." After all, these were people who were kind enough to call me, and I didn't want to make them feel uncomfortable. But even if I had no choice, the civilized world doesn't expect you to come right out and reveal all. My optimistic answers seemed to make most of my callers happy. I would have felt the same if I had made the call.

But sometimes, when the optimist failed to ask further about my health, I felt the impulse to attack. "Glad to hear you're doing so well," said one caller in response to my "reasonably well." He followed this with half an hour of his own suffering—"I'm in terrible shape"—and ending with, "Well, hope you keep improving. Bye-bye!" Sometimes being attentive seemed like an opportunity to even things up. There were those who responded to my cautious expressions of hope with reports about others who are doing badly. "That guy I work with, the one I was telling you about recently, he's going downhill fast." That was—I think—meant to give me a sense of relative privilege, but it felt like a dig. "Have I done something to hurt you?" I wondered.

Most callers are friendly and are prepared to listen, yet there are very few who give you the opportunity to go into detail. "There's still an abscess in my abdominal cavity." "Oh, really? But the main problem is okay, right? And that's great!" At first I used the word "infection" in my reports, but that led to discussions about boils. I tried to explain things by way of nuance but soon realized it was hopeless. It was too much for my caller to take on board. There aren't many people who like to hear about the kind of suffering that can affect them as well. By way of distraction they often came out with "I bet you're doing a lot of reading" or "Music must be doing you a world of good" or "Have you taken up painting again?" Art as life buoy.

One caller repeatedly took a far too rose-colored view of my situation, and finally I let him have it. I told him how badly things had gone the night before, how I had woken in a pile of shit and—leaving a trail behind me—had trudged to the bathroom to clean myself up as best I could and then to replace my equipment. "Thank God I can't smell very well, but it wasn't a pretty sight." Silence. "I hope things are going well for you. Bye!"

After a while I got a better grasp of how far I could go with my callers, those who only wanted "reasonably well" as an answer, those who always had a question about something else, those who only wanted to hear about the medical aspect of my ailment and nothing about the ailment itself. The callers who got furthest with me asked how all those tubes running into my body worked. But rarely was I able to tell my callers anything about cancer and excrement. Nor would I have wanted to do such a thing. Sick people have to become notoriously forgetful just to stay alive.

I myself am not a whit better than my callers. A famous Dutch journalist Renate Rubinstein wrote, "I wouldn't have called myself either."

I still feel guilty about dead people whom I failed to contact at the end of their lives. When I bumped into people who knew them I questioned them thoroughly. But call the person myself? No way. Even writing was difficult for me. Often I managed to send an umpteenth version of a note, but if I got no response I let it go at that. They've been dead for years and I still feel remorse, also because I was quite aware of the fact that I almost never wrote back. Being ill quickly makes you arrogant. "Making inquiries is for other people," is apparently what I thought.

Being sick is all right as long as it doesn't get too close. When that happens, callers switch to letters. They prefer to remain in control. They let me know they were thinking of me. Some of them wrote that they had read something I had written and very much appreciated it. The solace of a job well done. Apparently we're less restrained with our praise when the end is in sight. People start looking for the positive. But some people were so shocked by the word "cancer" that they thought I'd be gone in no time. They wrote farewell letters, accompanied by reflections on the inevitability of death. A Western man doesn't die without philosophy.

* * *

When sociologists do research on the networks of the sick, the relationships are scored on the basis of "contact or no contact" and "reciprocal or not reciprocal." Consequently, at the extreme ends of the scale there are two types: "unceasing help" and "disappearance of former acquaintances."

Much less research is conducted on what actually happens in those changing relationships. The vision of network sociologists is too detached for that. If they were less distant, they would discover the "optimism of illness" that sick people experience in their contacts. These are pleasant experiences for the sick if they proceed from a resistance to future suffering. They are less pleasant if they proceed from a compulsion to be optimistic, or if they prevent the sick from sharing their pain and pessimism.

The Silence of Illness

Medical sociologists do research on the experiences of the sick, usually by questioning sick people themselves. The sick are invited to come in and talk, mostly in somewhat artificial settings: in interviews with relative strangers. Another emerging kind of research involves direct conversations between doctors and patients, although it is limited to the health care system. So discussing what we know something about is done either by invitation or within the context of professional relationships. Talking about illness in everyday life, or choosing not to talk about it, is rarely a subject of this research.

So not only do sociologists hear what people have to say mainly by means of officially organized exchanges, but they also don't know what sick people are being silent about. When sociologists study conversations alone, all they hear is the official language of the doctor's office. They may notice that patients sometimes find it difficult to discuss certain things with their doctors—delicate subjects, for instance. But in this research method, what goes unsaid cannot be accessed. It can only be ascertained when the sick break their own silence. That is the advantage of studying the life stories of the sick.[1] People are more likely to talk freely in that type of research setting than in structured interviews. But even in a life story, a sick person may choose to remain silent.

Other people may also choose not to talk, such as those who meet with the sick. But that is something that sick sociologists can tell us about. They can reveal what others refuse to discuss.

* * *

If I can believe what I've been told, in all the time I've been sick I've never looked as good as I do now. There have been many who, upon meeting me, hastened to tell me how great I looked. Only one person added "but of course that's what they all say." He felt my suspicion.

I'm not the only one this has happened to. My hospital roommate had the same experience. No one looked bad, and apparently many looked unexpectedly good. There was never a lengthy conversation on this topic, however. Most people thought they had said quite enough about their sick friend with this one laudatory comment. The most extreme came from a couple who were visiting my roommate, a man who had been operated on a few days before. They entered the room with "my, you're looking well" and launched into an hour-long, impenetrable exchange about their daughter whom they had just visited in England and who had taken possession of an absolutely amazing house. All that time my roommate lay there with his debilitating condition, appearing to lend a friendly ear to everything they had to say.

When that aesthetic judgment is made of the person's appearance, paired with the lengthy stories, something "happens." These are "speech acts." The statement "my, you're looking well," for example, places the illness "offside." In my case it deprived me of my sickness. After such a judgment was made, the sickness was no longer part of the conversation. The statement was a license to move on to the order of the day, to ordinary life, because there was no longer anything unusual that we could have talked about.

Apparently most people prefer to hold illness at arm's length. That's why I, too, was regarded as "healthy" in interactions with outsiders. It wasn't that people were hassling me and expecting me to snap out of it and get back to normal. They were very circumspect in the way they treated me and eager to relieve me of my burdens. But there was little discussion of my illness. And as long as I didn't talk about what couldn't be seen, what was hidden behind the curtains of my clothing, they were quite prepared to believe what I said about everything being "fine."

People don't intend to hurt the sick. So what are they actually doing? I suspect that most of them think they're cheering the sick person up, or taking his mind off his worries. Others think they're helping him by pointing out how resilient the human body is. Most people, I believe, think that by flattering the sick person they're improving his mood. They feel sorry for the person, but they aren't very good at communicating it. They show that they're interested, and while they praise your appearance they're not oblivious to your ailment, although they keep it short. I myself usually found that was the best approach. You felt encouraged, and any attempt at nuance would only dampen that feeling. The sick person likes to hear that he's doing well and that other people are pleased with how he's doing. The opening statement was a starting point for something else, and I was all too willing to believe it myself.

But "you're looking well" can also be irritating. Why don't they want to know how things are going? Why am I not allowed to explain anything? There were very few people who wanted to know more about my condition, and only two or three who asked what exactly had been done to me. I still remember how eager I was to tell them: my blow-by-blow account of the operation and the hemorrhaging, and my detailed description of the two days of unconsciousness. And I was even more colorful in my explanation of the tubes attached to my body: one for the wound discharge, one for the urine, one for the infection, and one for my colostomy bag. When I stood in front of the mirror I looked like an astronaut under construction, I said with a strange sort of pride. But usually the questions were limited, and so were my answers. Almost no one wanted to hear about the excrement and the urine, about the pus from my intestines. And not a single soul was ready for my anxiety about departing this life. But I wasn't the only one to feel that fear. They, too, were afraid of being confronted by death.

I often had the feeling that it was better not to talk about my problems at all. The worst was behind me. Now the good old future was dawning again. And not even dawning. The future was already here. I almost looked like my old self, at least with my clothes on. So I really *was* my old self. The illness was over and done with, and I could resume my normal life, or at least that's what I thought they were thinking.

But their "looking well" deprived me of my legitimation to act like a sick person. The right to appeal to my illness was taken from me. "You look well, so why should I keep granting you the privileges of the sick?" That's what I thought they were thinking. Disqualified, that's how I sometimes felt. Silenced. If the illness was gone, on what grounds would I be able to refrain from doing anything? "My, you're looking well" sounded to me like a clean bill of health. Sometimes I had the barbaric inclination to tell such people that my mother, who had the same illness that I had down to the minutest detail, looked very well, too, on the day she died. Sometimes I sort of lost control and was struck by the urge to drop my trousers and show them what the "nether regions" actually looked like.

Of course I laughed along with them. I told them it was going better. But some days were better than others, I would hesitantly add. The more experienced I got as a sick person, the more reckless I became. I told them that with my particular illness you didn't necessarily look bad anyway, or that it all had to do with the weather.

Despite all the talk about illness on TV, our conversations about it are still quite limited. We speak cheerfully of the bypass operation that we happened to catch the evening before, but when talking to people who have had such an operation we still prefer to chat about football.

* * *

For a sociologist, it's not so interesting merely to note that when sick people are told "my, you're looking well" they are being both repudiated and ignored, and that fear of illness and death limits conversation. For an empirical sociologist, the interest lies in trying to determine how that happens, how "cheerfulness" forces illness from ordinary speech, for example, or how talking makes a sick person—as a sick person—persona non grata. A cheerful negation of the illness robs the sick person of his status. Compliments are used to suggest that the sick person either join the everyday world of the healthy or withdraw into the world of the sick.

People do not do this deliberately. They would be outraged to be accused of such a thing. The speaker is not the one who charges his words with meaning but the person being spoken to. And if that person is weaker, then that weak position becomes the message. The message I derived from all those compliments was not "don't bother me with your illness." The message was "the illness is gone." By complimenting me, the others could move on to their own agenda, or so I thought if I happened to be feeling defiant.

Being ill can continue unimpeded if it is "real" for people, if the sick person is visibly ill, if he is actually bedridden. The healthy-looking sick person has more difficulty. In his autobiography about his life with paraplegia, the anthropologist Robert Murphy wrote that when he was in the hospital people visited him, but when he was back at work they avoided him. After returning to work it's hard for the sick to carve out a place for themselves in day-to-day interactions.

Illness is socially regulated, with laws for sickness and disability benefits, with tests, company doctors, and insurance doctors. In that society, being sick is dominated not by the "medical regime" but by the "social regime." Once a sick person is officially recognized as ill by a doctor, we know what is expected of us in official terms: we are not to hold the person responsible for his own illness, and we are to excuse him from his duties. But in terms of informal, everyday existence, illness is still relatively unregulated. It's as if we were more comfortable excluding the sick from the order of the day. Sick people are better off exempting themselves from everyday life.

Frequently the sick just let it pass. They keep their ailments to themselves and don't talk about how they feel or what they are no longer able to do. Illness is for the bedroom and the bathroom, for places where people can be alone. The same goes for the family and friends of the sick: they, too, prefer to remain silent. A "health law" for everyday life has yet to be developed.

Illness is still an area of vulnerability in the life of a human being. Sociologists know this without having to do any research. But the fact that it is also a "sore spot" in society, a place where caution reigns, is something that sociologists are barely aware of. We say something similar about dying. We know that death takes place behind the scenes, even in isolation, says Norbert Elias (1985). But perhaps not anymore. I know some people who broke their vow of silence at that very moment and were able to speak, sometimes for the first time.

All too often we think that illness is a frequent topic of conversation. That may be true in the case of temporary ailments. We could probably talk for hours on end about a broken leg. But when it comes to life-threatening illnesses there's more a sense of taboo. The same is true of mental illnesses, which is why people suffering from depression sometimes wish they had a broken leg. When illness strikes we hope—preferably in silence—that everything will come out all right, and we're all too happy with the smallest sign of improvement. Not only because things are going well, but also for our own spiritual welfare. If things go badly, we prefer to remain silent. The isolation of illness is not that people stay away. The isolation of illness can be found in the refusal to talk, in the "silence of illness."

Keeping Silent

When sociologists conduct interviews, they usually focus on the talk and rarely on the silence. We know that people are silent about a great many things, but it's their talking that we listen to. It's true that we encourage them to talk, but the things that people keep their mouths shut about escape us. Some sociologists believe they have come up with something to deal with this problem: the depth interview. This gives them more of a story, but not the story that people are usually silent about, or the story they only think about, or don't think about at all, or the story about what people only do. That's why sociologists who ask questions are often unaware of what illness means for sick people, of what sick people do themselves.

In medical sociology, illness appears mainly in two forms: first, as a physical fact as "seen" by doctors and as "seen" by sick people in the language of the sick. In research having to do with this first form, the illness has already been described by others. These sociologists are only interested in the external aspects of the illness: the social causes of the illness, for example, or its social consequences, or the experiences people have with such an illness. In such research, what the sick have to say is subordinate to the illness itself. The focus is on the illness, and the interview is all about that illness. Talking is a marginal event.

All this changes when illness is seen as an ongoing construct that is made up of practices, especially linguistic practices. Construction also takes place in the first approach, but it is less evident. Because the doctor's linguistic construct is ideologically dominant, the illness appears to be something that simply *is* rather than the product of the doctor's language, i.e. of medical interpretation. Construct research is therefore mainly focused on the sick. The assumption is that the sick have their own view of what is affecting them, which is often different from that of the doctors.

But in both approaches, the "silent illness" remains unspoken: the illness that lurks only in the heads of the sick, the illness that is suppressed, to which not a single word is devoted, the illness that is hidden from language, the illness that at the very most lends itself to action but not to language.

The only sociologists who try to get to the bottom of these silences are the ones with good eyes, the ones who observe, the ethnographers. But there is one other category of sociologists who are also very good at understanding silence: sociologists who themselves are ill. For a while I was such a sociologist.

* * *

Illness brings out the best in people. They let me know that they sympathized with me. They wished me the best, gave me hope, talked about people with the same illness who were doing well, and gave me lots of advice, especially about food. Nor did my lifestyle go unmentioned. People asked me a great many questions: how I was doing, how I felt and whether I noticed any improvement, whether I was still able to pass the time meaningfully, and whether I felt like living anymore.

What very few of them asked, however, was what the operation had entailed, what the surgeons had done to me, and how my body was functioning after all that radical surgery. No one said a thing about the tubes that had been connected to my body. Although people knew I had had a colostomy—most of them seemed to have heard it from others—only two asked how something like that works. Sometimes I tried to explain it myself, but I soon stopped. It didn't take long to realize that this was not a comfortable topic of conversation.

What cannot be seen, what is only seen in hospital rooms, and then by "privileged" witnesses alone, what even confidantes only hear about, there the sick play their own linguistic games. The others sometimes share what they think they know within their own circles. A great deal remains unsaid, suspected at the most, and quickly forgotten or suppressed. Often the decision is made to just let things pass. Under such linguist conditions, the sick feel the community of silence.

This was not unexpected. Who likes to talk about the decomposition of the body, about chances of survival, or about confrontations with death? Who is eager to ask about the body's waste disposal system? And who enjoys hearing descriptions of disposal system accidents? I wouldn't have wanted to listen to myself either.

* * *

The words that rattle around inside the head, or bounce off the walls of empty rooms, or are reduced to gestures or fiddling about in little compartments, these things turn illness into a "backstage phenomenon." That backstage setting is something we ourselves create. There are peepholes backstage that give the sick a glimpse of society, a view of others, people who prefer to pay no attention to what is going on behind the scenes.

Being silent is not so unusual. There are many things that we hardly ever talk about: about anxiety and depression, about how much we detest certain people, about envy and jealousy, about what went wrong, or what is beyond reach, or what we are ashamed of, and so much more.

When it comes to public display we get the opposite impression: we watch bloody operations in great detail on TV, we see people crying on Oprah because they've neglected their children, others discuss their marital hopes for all the world to see, people have sex as if they were actors, we rush to the sites of accidents, people curse and swear about private matters in public. But in our daily existence all that openness is limited. Illness, if it's serious, falls under the regime of silence. Where illness is, silence reigns.

That silence distances the sick from others, and others from them. Sick people have something that others would rather not mention in everyday discourse. Illness is often a topic of conversation, but mainly in terms of the name of the disease and rarely in conversations with the sick person himself. Conversational circles pop up around him.[2] There information is exchanged and judgments are made, explanations are voiced and predictions aired. But little from those circles makes it way to the sick. They live within the "silence of illness," surrounded by noise.

The reason sociologists have rarely written about this silence is because they are mainly interested in linguistic approaches. Their chief research method is the interview. But even when they are observing, silence and taciturnity are difficult to interpret. In order to realize that something is not being talked about, and to discover what it is, they have to know what's going on. The best way to learn about this is to be sick oneself.

Silences usually indicate discomfort and uncertainty. They concern something that is best left unsaid. But not all absence of speech is silence. Silence can also go unnoticed because it's appropriate to the situation. Silences can be noiseless but they can also be full of sound, as when someone "changes the subject." Choosing not to speak can go hand-in-hand with a great deal of linguistic noise.

In our society, remaining silent is a moral act. Usually we are required to speak the truth. Silence and the decision not to speak are inappropriate in many interactions. It's important to keep the conversation going. If you call someone and he doesn't say anything, you become irritated (Silverman 1998: 10). That explains the moral battle that is fought on the question of deliberate silence. The indignation that arises when something does not come up for discussion can take grotesque forms. But most of the time it is expressed indirectly and later on. Silences are peepholes on the morality of society. They show us what is inappropriate, what is based on taboo, what must remain hidden. This is how conversation analysts track down the rules of conversation, such as the rule that silence in response to a question asked by a judge during an interrogation indicates "doubt" or "a lie" (Silverman 1998: 10).

Silence and the refusal to speak turn illness into a moral phenomenon, something you can't say just anything about. The refusal to speak turns illness into a precarious social situation, something that must be approached with great caution. When people are speaking with a sick person about his illness, they can't just blurt out whatever comes into their heads. And a sick person cannot say anything he wants to, either. Not only does the morality of illness keep people from speaking, but, conversely, the refusal to speak makes illness a moral phenomenon.

That moral aspect is what makes it so difficult to relate to sick people. What do you say to them, and when? What topics do you bring up later on? What do you keep under wraps? Why haven't you said it yet? Why don't you say anything else? Why didn't you seize the opportunity? And then there's the reassurance. It's better for the sick person not to have known. Talking about it would only have disturbed him. Plenty of reasons for a good solid sociological study.

Notes

1. In my research on images of chronic illnesses I make use of life stories. For the method of life stories, see Scott (1990), Rosenwald and Ochberg (1992), Lieblich and Josselson (1997), Millar (2000), Smith and Watson (2001), Anderson (2001), and Czarniawska (2004).
2. Sometimes they create their own discussion groups with empathetic people who have experience with the illness. Monks (1995) discovered such groups in her study of people with MS. She called them "MS talk" groups.

References

Anderson, L. 2001. *Autobiography.* London: Routledge.

Berg, M. 1992. The Construction of Medical Disposals. *Sociology of Health & Illness* 14: 151–180.

Czarniawska, B. 2004. *Narratives in Social Science Research.* London: Sage.

De Swaan, A. 1990. *The Management of Normality.* London and New York: Routledge.

Elias, N. 1985. *The Loneliness of the Dying.* Oxford: Basil Blackwell.

Fox, R. 1959. *Experiment Perilous: Physicians and Patients Facing the Unknown.* New York: The Free Press of Glencoe.

Glaser, B., and A. Strauss. 1965. *Awareness of Dying.* Chicago: Aldine.

Goffman, E. 1959. *The Presentation of Self in Everyday Life.* New York: Anchor Books.

Lieblich, A., and R. Josselson (eds.). 1997. *The Narrative Study of Life.* Thousand Oaks: Sage.

Millar, R. 2000. *Researching Life Stories and Family Histories.* London: Sage.

Monks, J. 1995. Life Stories and Sickness Experience. *Culture, Medicine and Psychiatry* 19: 453–478.

Rosenwald, G., and R. Ochberg (eds.). 1992. *Storied Lives.* New Haven: Yale University Press.

Scott, J. 1990. *A Matter of Record.* London: Polity Press.

Silverman, D. 1998. *Harvey Sacks: Social Science and Conversational Analysis.* Cambridge: Polity Press.

Smith, S., and J. Watson. 2001. *Reading Autobiography.* Minneapolis: University of Minnesota Press.

Sudnow, D. 1967. *Passing On: The Social Organization of Dying.* Englewood Cliffs: Prentice Hall.

The, A.-M. 2002. *Palliative Care and Communication: Experiences in the Clinic.* Buckingham: Open University Press.

CHAPTER 8

Legitimation

Abstract Patients feel insecure. Their body has betrayed them. Many patients not only lose trust in themselves; the world as a whole becomes suspect and strange. It is easy to get sick, but not easy to be sick. Illness pushes people "out of place." Fortunately, there is the sick role, which legitimates their deviant behavior. If people know about my sickness, they will excuse me when I fail in what is expected of me. Illness is made up of interpretations, but usually it's a healthy person who directs the interpretation. The aim of sociologists should be to figure out how sick people and their surroundings turn the illness into what it becomes socially. Serious illness is a voyage into the unknown. The world becomes a place for deliberation.

Keywords Unreliability · Legitimation work · Sociology · Illness as construct

Unreliability

The uncertainty of the sick has been a much-researched topic in the annals of medical sociology. Usually this research has to do with uncertainty about the future development of the illness, about what the sick person will still be able to do, and about the future of life with the illness. There has been far less research on ongoing uncertainty, on the uncertainty that the illness triggers in your life.

G. Nijhof, *Sickness Work*,
https://doi.org/10.1007/978-981-13-0326-5_8

Illness doesn't just change your life. It also increases the uncertainty you feel about what is going to change in your life and what isn't. That uncertainty is difficult for the sick person but it's especially difficult for others, which makes it even more difficult for the sick person himself—not because the uncertainty of others makes him feel even more uncertain, but because his uncertainty makes him unreliable. Someone who is uncertain becomes unpredictable, and that unpredictability affects his reliability. Sick people cannot be counted on. They don't know if they'll be able to do tomorrow what they could still do today, so others don't know it either. In this way illness becomes a "reliability problem."

Trust is the cement that holds society together. Of course there are unreliable people. Of course we don't trust what some people do. And our trust is regularly being shaken. But by and large we trust the world around us as a matter of course, as if it were normal, "natural." We trust that the busses will run on time and that people will do what they've always done. We count on bread being available tomorrow, on partners coming home when they say they're going to town, on people being hungry if they say they're hungry, on being ill if they're told they're ill, and we trust people not to deceive us if they say they feel well.

Shaking people's trust is seen as a serious offense. Such people go down in our estimation. We tell them that we "hadn't expected that of them," often adding, "especially not of them." People bear the stigma of unreliability for a long time. The accusation of unreliability can even become part of their profile. Shaken trust is something we do not take lightly.

Shaking people's trust is not just a matter of doing something unexpected. It's also a breach of social morality. People do not easily let it pass. Society doesn't run by rules and role expectations alone. Society also demands predictability, and hence trust. If we could no longer trust anything or anyone, I believe we'd all go mad.

Many sick people seem to lose faith in themselves. People with Parkinson's disease, for example, not only lose faith in their bodies (what they used to take for granted is now a cause of uncertainty), but they also lose faith in themselves—their self-confidence is undermined. And both these things make their world unreliable; they have to rediscover what they used to take for granted in their former world (cf., Nijhof 1996).

Sick people experience the opposite of that trust. They notice that they are less trusted by others. But not only that. They also notice that other people sometimes find them less reliable.

* * *

From all appearances nothing in my life seems to have changed. People who haven't heard don't see anything different about me. They talk to me about the ordinary, everyday things of life. But I have my reservations. Isn't it better that I tell them something? I could be admitted to the hospital at any time. And there are still complications, which sometimes result in unexpected behavior. Maybe something should be done to deal with that? Maybe I should have another operation? But then I wouldn't be able to do what I've just promised to do. What's even more difficult is that my condition is sometimes unpredictable. I can feel fine one minute and tired the next, able to do very little. Sometimes I feel so good that I become overconfident. It's going to get even better in the future, I say to myself. But then suddenly something happens, and the predictions for the future have to be re-adjusted. Is this something I always have to keep in mind? Should I inform everyone who is dependent on me? Are things going to get better tomorrow, or not?

My best relationships are with people who know me, of course, such as my colleagues. One of those colleagues could see things were headed in the wrong direction even before I knew it myself. She took over my teaching load. But would I be able to teach my course the following trimester? I thought so. But the recovery was slower than expected, and once again the same colleague saw before I did that it wouldn't be possible and took over for me. The next academic year I was sure I'd be able to do all my work myself. But suddenly I found out that I had to have yet another operation. The only possible time was in the middle of the trimester. Once again, colleagues offered to take over my four remaining teaching weeks. "Will that be all?" I thought they'd be asking themselves. The situation with my students was also precarious. Could I really subject them to unforeseeable interruptions in the supervision of their theses?

Uncertainty also struck in my private life. Could I go on vacation? Hesitation. Decision postponed. Yet finally I was talked into deciding. Hadn't I ever heard of cancellation insurance? And planes to fly me back home? I gave in, but insisted on a nearby country, just in case. And could I go to my daughter's party? Yes, I thought. Three days in London should be possible. But after one operation my decision soon proved untenable. Party postponed.

All that unpredictability made me feel increasingly unreliable. After breaking one agreement I promised more than I could deliver. That felt even more unreliable. The people around me understood that when I explained it to them, and didn't blame me personally. But in my head it's different. There I'm an unreliable skunk who does whatever works best for him. The English sociologist Ruth Pinder put it better than I could: for others it isn't "business as usual" but "think specially." She must have been ill herself, I thought when I read that. She hadn't been. But her husband has Parkinson's disease. She observed it in the life of another.

My wife had the most trouble with uncertainty. She noticed it in almost everything we did. She knew, even if I didn't say so, that I felt uncertain. That is the daily problem of living with a sick person, living with someone who is unsure of so much, keeps away from many things, postpones decisions, says that it's better to wait until he's sure about when something can happen, until he's experienced how the body will respond after an operation. But for others it's hard to tell the difference between holding back and being obstinate. This is the field in which unreliability flourishes.

My hemming and hawing makes Mar even more decisive. "Should I make restaurant reservations?" "We can always cancel, you know." "Should I buy tickets for the theater?" "If you can't manage it, we won't go." "But we *are* going to Mali, right?" And there I am, hesitating and raising objections. "Do you think they have hotel rooms with baths in Mali?" "I still have that infection." "The stoma still has to be finished off." And "you see how tired I can get from one minute to the next, so I can hardly do anything." My spluttering never stops.

But every time we do something it goes better than expected. We go to a movie or to the theater, we go on vacation, we take bike trips to places that haven't been part of our cycling repertoire in recent years as far as I can remember. We do much more than I thought I could do. But that, too, makes me unreliable, I think.

Sometimes I'm overtaken by euphoria. I keep saying over and over again how wonderful it is that I can do a particular thing once more. That I had never thought it possible. But once we get home I start thinking, "What if I were to get sick somewhere?" "Can I sleep in a tent?" Uncertainty strikes again, and with it unreliability.

Uncertainty is difficult to dispel. I myself have learned to live with it. I believe I have good reasons for my hesitation, and if I have them, I hide them—behind piles of work, for example. But those who live with me have to deal with a hesitant procrastinator, with someone who smells of unreliability.

* * *

Trust is what makes it possible for us to take the world for granted. Of course we can't always do that, but when we can't it's usually because something has gone wrong. Maybe something has happened. Maybe someone has been careless. Maybe someone has been malicious. When people behave in an unconventional way we expect excuses, and then order is restored. But if a person's behavior becomes erratic and chronic, if what once was taken for granted must now be spelled out, then unreliability becomes the leaven that permeates relationships with him.

So if we can't tell what sick people are going to do next, that makes them not only unpredictable but also unreliable. Unpredictability makes the sick unreliable. And that unreliability makes them deviant. They become a stick in the wheel of everyday life. The sick challenge our belief that we can take everyday life for granted. They upset the idea of "business as usual." The sick cannot be counted on. Their unreliability becomes a problem, which makes them feel unreliable. So to be ill is to live a life of unreliability, and living with a sick person means living with unreliability.

This also makes illness a problem of interaction. The sick are socially problematic individuals. Because they are unreliable, they occupy the same life category as criminals, the insane, and the fickle.

Sociologists have long known that, socially speaking, illness is not just illness. In the fifties, the sociologist Parsons imputed deviant behavior to the sick and saw it as one of the greatest threats to our Western social order. If people were to work only when they wanted to, and if they were to stop working whenever they saw fit, our economic order would quickly disintegrate. For this reason he saw illness as the most threatening reason that people could advance for their own deviant behavior. Consequently, people should not be allowed to declare themselves "ill." If this responsibility were borne by doctors alone, the functioning of the economic order would be saved. This, he wrote, is the best idea to be produced by medical sociology.

Our society controls this deviance by allowing doctors the exclusive right to hand down the verdict. Only professional physicians may decide if people are too ill to work. This serves to regulate the deviance and removes the odor of unreliability from non-working people. Their deviant behavior has been officially confirmed, and legitimized, by doctors.

But this medical endorsement plays a much less important role outside the realm of employment. There both the sick and the healthy have to work things out among themselves. There people are forced to rely on their own "good will" and that of others, which makes for a precarious relationship. So being ill is a shaky existence, and the odor of unreliability soon returns.

Legitimation Work

It's easy to get sick, but not easy to be sick. That is because, as previously noted, illness undermines society. And that in turn is becausesystem is too incidental those who are sick are allowed to give up doing certain things, which quickly endangers the social order. Within this social order it has been agreed that everyone will fulfill their everyday obligations and earn their living by working, unless they are not able to do so or unless all the rest of us come to the conclusion that we cannot (or can no longer) expect it of them. So abandoning your obligations and not working is not something that is easily done, and one of the few excuses that we are prepared to accept is illness. For sick people there is the sick role, which legitimates their deviant behavior. This sick role is an ingenious discovery.

Work is surrounded by guarantees. Workers themselves are not free to decide whether to work or not. That would make society unstable. For this reason, rules are put in place to curb absenteeism, and only certain grounds are accepted. Illness is one of those recognized grounds. But even this ground is not left to the workers to manage themselves. Doctors are called into assess the presence of illness. The requirement of a doctor's certificate signifies social control. This process of social control has become institutionalized in the sick role.

People who are allotted this role are given certain rights, but they may only exercise those rights if they also assume certain obligations. The first obligation is to find the status of sick person undesirable, with the concomitant obligation being to make an effort to get better by seeking the help of official healthcare workers and by cooperating with them. You can't just merrily call the office and say you don't feel like working so you're calling in sick. You must tell your employer, with a cheerless voice, that you are ill and you are not able to work. But that's not enough. You employer is not going to take you at your word. The ailment must be recognized as a genuine "illness" by a doctor. Only a doctor has the authority to do this. He can verify whether someone can justifiably feel himself exempted from his obligations. A sick person is also required to seek competent help, also from a doctor. Only when all this has been done can you claim your rights, according to the sick role theory. There are two such rights. The first is the right to be released from normal obligations. The second is that although the illness is be regarded as deviant behavior, people are not to be held responsible for getting sick and therefore cannot be expected to get better by their own efforts. In this sick role, people can justifiably feel exempt from their obligations. Sick people can then rightfully and reasonably say that they are "ill" and know that their illness is socially accepted.

People who are chronically ill can also make use of this sick role, especially if the illness has only recently manifested itself. But if the ailment goes on for a longer period of time it is often difficult to tell whether they can continue to claim the right to be treated like a sick person. Their condition is not temporary, while the sick role is geared towards temporary exemption. This raises the question, especially for them, as to whether they can continue to lay claim to the legitimation offered by the role of an acute sufferer. Apparently this legitimation applies to a lesser degree to the chronically ill and disabled. And that is a problem because other sources of justification that are as unquestioned as the sick role are not available to them.

* * *

When I talk about my ailments, my operation, and the aftereffects thereof, I talk mainly to myself and the people I'm close to. That's not really a problem for me. I'm used to keeping a great deal to myself. It only became a problem when I started getting better, especially for those who didn't really know what was wrong with me, or what kinds of demands the illness made on the way I organized my daily existence, or whether the illness was keeping me from doing things that others took for granted. Most people remember that I cannot eat everything, and they take the necessary measures. But when I started looking normal and still said there were things I couldn't do, it became more difficult—for others and consequently for me as well. And if I'm late for an appointment because my colostomy bag has suddenly begun leaking, it's also problematic. My excuse is exactly what people don't want to hear about.

So if I make something up, there's the inconvenience. If I suddenly get tired and excuse myself, I'm afraid it will be seen as shirking my duties. And if I leave a meeting twice in quick succession to do something in the bathroom, I worry that others are thinking that the conversation doesn't please me. If people don't know what I'm dealing with, the things I take for granted are not the same as theirs.

Things unsaid lead to uncertainty. If people are uninformed, they make up their own theories. "Yesterday he was doing fine and today he says he can't go a step further. It must be unwillingness, or aversion, or indifference, or arrogance, or negligence." People don't actually say that, I think. Silence means I don't know what they're thinking, and they don't know how I'm doing. As a result, my life with this illness is split into a world of talk and a world of silence. In the former world people know me, in the latter world they don't. People in the world of silence have no explanation for my behavior. That makes me unpredictable in the eyes of others, or maybe even unreliable. At least that's what I suspect. I'm not sure about how the behavior I reveal is being interpreted. I have difficulty making my behavior readily understood. If I sense that something is going wrong, I have a legitimation problem. Thus my world is twice surrounded: by silence and by my impression that I've become unreliable.

* * *

For people with chronic conditions there are hardly any specific roles that they can fall back on. The treatment they usually receive is so infrequent that they are unable to lay claim to the position of "patient." Their contact with the healthcare system is too incidental. People with a chronic condition are usually not so ill that they can occupy the "sick role" for a long period of time. If they aren't sick enough to qualify for the role of "disabled," they run the risk of falling into a role-less situation. This means they have no role at their disposal that is reserved just for them and is appropriate to their condition, a role they can legitimately adopt, a role they can appeal to whenever questions arise concerning their behavior. People with a chronic condition cannot take for granted the legitimation that the sick role offers to those with an acute illness.

So after a while, people with chronic conditions find themselves in a situation in which their ailment is no longer simply taken as legitimation of their deviant behavior. Adjustments are often made for them, and after the initial disruption the sick person appears to be living a relatively normal life. They can usually resume their social life to a limited extent, or their behavior gives people the impression that nothing serious is wrong. In addition, the signs of their condition are often invisible. In such a situation, it is difficult to accept an appeal to the ailment as grounds for exemption from duties. Others look at them with suspicion because it isn't clear why and to what extent their capacity to work has been affected. People wonder whether they have the right to claim special treatment. Sometimes their claim is openly challenged, but usually it never goes beyond a hidden wariness and a suspicion that the person himself is up to something.

People with chronic conditions find themselves in a semi-institutionalized social space. There is no "regulated" place in society that is open to them, which is why they risk running into legitimation problems. Because they have no access to generally recognized forms of legitimation, other people don't know how to identify them. And that jeopardizes the reliability of people with long-term illnesses.

This opens up a whole new area of sociological research with regard to the sick, in this case focused on the undiscussed, the implausible, and the unreliable. How does the silence occur? When things are talked about, how is the backstage constructed? How does the picture of unreliability arise in interpersonal exchanges? How do people with chronic conditions attempt to legitimize themselves? How do they explain their situation? How do they justify the things they do differently? What is the "dynamic of their disqualification"? And that of their legitimation?

Illness as Construct

From a sociological point of view, the social reality of illness is "made" in word and gesture. Of course there is the body. But illness presents itself to others and to the sick person himself in terms of signs. Which signs? From whom? And of what? And how are these signs to be interpreted? How are the signs of the body to be "read"? And how are we to read the signs made by doctors concerning the signs of the body?

These questions explain why illness often assumes different forms in our social lives. The interpretations of the sick often change. They may take no notice of something that only recently they had attached their fate to. Sometimes they're hopeful, and sadness is out of the question. At other times they lose hope and stare vacantly into space. Most of the time, however, their lives are dominated by goodness. Sick people usually exhibit positive traits in the books they write about themselves and that others write about them, and bravery is at the top of the list.

* * *

Illness is made up of interpretations, but usually it's a healthy person who's asking the questions. "How are you doing?" I didn't know myself how I was doing most of the time. Yesterday it wasn't so great. Today I feel somewhat better. How do you answer such a question? "I feel fine," I heard myself say. But at the same time I was thinking, "That doctor did look a bit worried just now." What is a valid answer? If my answers vary, does that mean I'm unreliable? And if I don't say what I'm thinking, am I being a hypocrite?

And then there's the questioner. Answers are usually formulated with an audience in mind. Some questioners would rather hear a cheerful answer, I thought, because it frees them from having to deal with a lot of difficulties. There are other questioners with whom I had never previously shared much personal information, so why do it now? And then there were others who weren't in very good shape themselves. Why burden them with my tales of woe? And with others I just didn't want to be a complainer; I'd rather be someone who toughs it out.

No two conversations were the same, either in content or in tone. I told one person things were going very well, and another that while there was progress it was all happening very slowly. I told yet another that I was afraid things were not going well at all, now that I knew more about my limited chances. In one conversation I talked mostly about the side issues such as back pain, as if that had been the reason for my operation. And in another I concentrated on the operation that was coming up next, apparently to keep them from thinking that it was all behind me, that I was back to "business as usual." One person asked so many questions that I began to get defensive and adjusted my answers accordingly. Another wanted to talk mainly about the nuts and bolts of the operation, and I grabbed the opportunity to go into great detail. I didn't get very many chances like that, and I talked non-stop. In another case I felt ashamed because I didn't even have the answers to her questions, questions I hadn't dared ask my doctor.

* * *

Being ill is a linguistic game. Answers are continually offered to suit the person and the situation, the hour of the day and the condition, the mood and the state of mind, what has happened and what is yet to come.

Sociologists are trained to ask people questions, so many of them expect to get answers. And there are even those who think the answer is already in their brain, fully-formed and waiting to be uttered. Such sociologists think that a sick person knows how he is doing, that all he has to do is disclose it whenever he is asked to do so. As if there were such a thing as a state of being ill, a state that a sick person can talk about reliably and with valid answers. Such sociologists think that being ill is like an illness, something that can simply be diagnosed. It's either there or it isn't. It has a certain shape and only has to be revealed.

For some sociologists, illness is hidden in interpretation, in what is said about it. For other sociologists, being ill is mainly an interactional construction, a product of contact. In such cases, the answer to a question about the sick person's condition is "good" if it turns out there's not much to say about the illness, or if the sick person doesn't want to distress the questioner. The answer is "bad" if the other is expected to be able to do something about it, or for God knows what other reason.

Rather than joining the chorus of questioners, sociologists would be better off studying the kinds of things a sick person says to the people he comes in contact with. And studying what the others say in response. And back and forth again. They should not limit themselves to questions about how the sick person "is." In the social realm, nothing *is*. Everything is constructed on site, in local interpretations. The aim of sociologists is to figure out how sick people and their questioners turn the illness into what it becomes socially. Sometimes they turn the illness into a relationship that can be tolerated by both parties. Sometimes they screen themselves off, and both parties search for protection from the threat of calamity, keeping outsiders at bay, putting intruders in their place, refusing admission to those who give offense, and turning illness into a private phenomenon. Sometimes illness becomes a demand for attention, and the sick just string their sympathizers along. Sometimes illness becomes a form of intimacy.

Sociologically speaking, illness is whatever those who talk about it make of it, whatever they construct in their speech. Sociologically, illness is a social construct of that which, medically speaking, is called "illness."

Reference

Nijhof, G. 1996. Uncertainty and Lack of Trust with Parkinson's Disease. *European Journal of Public Health* 6 (1): 58–63.

CHAPTER 9

Epilogue

Abstract Looking back I realize that this book is not about emotions; it is about accepting illness—and the work it requires—as a normal part of life. Normal is what you do without thinking about it. This book is like a traveler's chronicle. Everything that had seemed exciting and unusual at first turned out to be quite ordinary after a brief stay. It is precisely because things become ordinary that society is possible.

Keywords Acceptance · Normality · Daily routine

This book has become quite different with the passing of time. In my rounds of revision I changed the present tense to the past tense in a few places, and sometimes vice versa. Every now and then I'd re-read a passage that struck me as cranky. Once problems are over they often seem minuscule. But even if they become permanent, or if certain limitations aren't evident until later on, it often felt to me as if I had been making a mountain out of a molehill. I appear to have gotten used to many of the things that were problematic at first. The limitations became part of my day-to-day life. It was still "different," but no longer anything to fret about. Complaints, ailments, and limitations just become the order of the day—until something goes wrong. Then the precautions and habituation start all over again.

As a sociologist I should have known that, of course. It's precisely because things become ordinary that a society is even possible, and

G. Nijhof, *Sickness Work*,
https://doi.org/10.1007/978-981-13-0326-5_9

because such an ordinary society exists, sociology also exists. Because we have the marvelous ability to integrate many things that happen to us over time and to regard them as ordinary, even to take them for granted, an order arises that appears natural to us. That natural order is the hard core of what we call society. It is through the "naturalization" of the world around us that the "hardware" of society is made.

Many people fight against this certainty: children who have little knowledge of the past, the elderly who feel that they've lost touch with their own naturalness, young people who look ahead to the fashion of tomorrow, politicians who think things should be different, sociologists who can't stop detecting change.

Every society has its own conservative forces, however, and it's because of them that something we can call "social" exists. If all we had was change, we wouldn't be able to understand each other, and every individual would lapse into madness. It was a sociologist of earlier times—Alfred Schutz—who reminded us of this. He wrote about the "natural attitude": our propensity to regard what we do and what surrounds us as ordinary and to take it for granted, to regard it as *the* reality. It is the capacity of the human species to make new things into old things, things we are used to, things we find ordinary, things we know nothing about except that they're self-evident. The beauty of this is that we don't have to learn about it in courses and therapy sessions. This naturalization is instilled in us through the mere act of living together. We are simply forced to get on with our lives.

It is this capacity that is so beneficial to people with chronic illnesses. Psychologists insist that illnesses should be processed, that people should take care to defend themselves from their suffering, that they should face up to their illness and the distress it causes. But sick people and sociologists can respond by arguing that the ailments, limitations, and impediments need to become ordinary, an aspect of their normal life—that they should become part of the bodily equipment that we take for granted.

The problem is that others tend to regard the ailment as normal before the sick person does. Those around him often slip back into the daily routine more readily. In the eyes of the sick person, these others no longer see what's going on. They're oblivious to it, they take no notice of it, and in doing so they ignore him and his limitations. This tendency to naturalize the life of the sick at different tempos is what tears them apart. But, like everything else, they get used to it.

That's why this book is not about emotions. It's about accepting illness—and the work it requires—as a normal part of life. Accepting something as normal doesn't just happen, if only because it's not just in your head. It's also a matter of doing. A thing is only normal if you do it without thinking about it. So this book is mainly about technique, about the work of learning to do unusual things in an ordinary way, about developing routines.

This is why the things I wrote about seemed to age so rapidly. No sooner had I learned something than it became normal, and writing about it was hardly worth the effort. That wasn't true when I first wrote about it, however, which is why I wrote about it in the first place.

Accepting one's own life as normal had its counterpart in having more understanding for others. My writing contained a lot of grumbling about other people. Apparently because I was ill, I counted on sympathy and help. But being ill is a precarious business that we have trouble relating to, not only when we ourselves are ill but also when the illness affects someone else. For both the sick and the healthy, illness reminds us of the fragility of existence. It upsets the idea of ordinary life that we take for granted: that mind and body are going to keep on going. For the sick that banal trust is shattered. Their life of illness is an implicit call to others to sympathize with that feeling. And many do, with courage and loyalty. But some people show their fear in distasteful and evasive behavior. I have taken that behavior for negligence, something I only now understand.

Anything a person might say about his life is always a current interpretation, even if it's a sick person's life story. Life stories are never descriptions of a life but are always interpretations of that life. And these interpretations are time-specific, not with respect to the time of the life but to the time of the telling. That, too, is why life stories that have been written down are so subject to ageing, at least for their authors. I had already considered that theoretically in my sociological studies in which I used life stories as a method. In the story of my own illness I experienced it firsthand.

So this book is like a traveler's chronicle. Everything that had seemed exciting and unusual at first turned out to be quite ordinary after a brief stay. After a few days I was willing to trade the most beautiful panoramic view for a book I could just as easily have read at home. After staring our eyes out at the people walking past us that first evening in Taroudant, I spent the next day at the same outdoor cafe talking about nothing in particular. And only a few days after having been astonished by the glories of Fez, I walked around as if I lived there and had no other need than fruit juice. Being ill is like traveling. You have lots of unusual experiences, but after a while you accept it all as perfectly normal.

Illness will never be completely normal, however. Raging below the surface is the fire of eventual death. I've looked over the edge of the ordinary and I've already forgotten what I saw there. But I did see something. And no society is going to take that away from me.

Bibliography

Alexander, L. 1981. The Double-Bind Between Dialysis Patients and Their Health Practitioners. In *The Relevance of Social Science for Medicine*, ed. L. Eisenberg and A. Kleinman, 307–329. Dordrecht, Boston, and London: Reidel.

Anderson, L. 2001. *Autobiography*. London: Routledge.

Berg, M. 1992. The Construction of Medical Disposals. *Sociology of Health and Illness* 14: 151–180.

Bury, M. 1982. Chronic Illness as Biographical Disruption. *Sociology of Health and Illness* 4: 167–182.

Calnan, M. 1984. Clinical Uncertainty: Is It a Problem in the Doctor–Patient Relationship? *Sociology of Health and Illness* 6: 74–85.

Caplan, G. 1964. *Principles of Preventive Psychiatry*. London: Tavistock.

Corbin, J., and A. Strauss. 1988. *Unending Work and Care: Managing Chronic Illness at Home*. San Francisco and London: Jossey-Bass.

Czarniawska, B. 2004. *Narratives in Social Science Research*. London: Sage.

De Swaan, A. 1990. *The Management of Normality*. London and New York: Routledge.

Elias, N. 1985. *The Loneliness of the Dying*. Oxford: Basil Blackwell.

Fox, R. 1959. *Experiment Perilous: Physicians and Patients Facing the Unknown*. New York: The Free Press of Glencoe.

Frank, A. 1991. *At the Will of the Body: Reflections on Illness*. Boston: Houghton Mifflin.

Frank, A. 2001. Can We Research Suffering? *Qualitative Health Research* 11 (3): 353–362.

Frank, A. 2004. After Methods, the Story: From Incongruity to Truth in Qualitative Research. *Qualitative Health Research* 14 (3): 430–440.

G. Nijhof, *Sickness Work*,
https://doi.org/10.1007/978-981-13-0326-5

French, S. 1993. 'Can You See the Rainbow?' The Roots of Denial. In *Disabling Barriers—Enabling Environments*, ed. J. Swain, et al., 69–77. London: Sage.

Garfinkel, H. 1967. *Studies in Ethnomethodology*. Englewood Cliffs: Prentice-Hall.

Glaser, B., and A. Strauss. 1965. *Awareness of Dying*. Chicago: Aldine.

Goffman, E. 1959. *The Presentation of Self in Everyday Life*. New York: Anchor Books.

Goffman, E. 1963. *Stigma, Notes on the Management of Spoiled Identity*. Englewood Cliffs: Prentice-Hall.

Heritage, J. 1984. *Garfinkel and Ethnomethodology*. Cambridge: Polity Press.

Kaufert, J., and D. Locker. 1990. Rehabilitation Ideology and Respiratory Support Technology. *Social Science & Medicine* 30 (8): 867–877.

Lefton, M. 1984. Chronic Disease and Applied Sociology: An Essay in Personalised Sociology. *Sociological Inquiry* 54: 466–476.

Lieblich, A., and R. Josselson (eds.). 1997. *The Narrative Study of Life*. Thousand Oaks: Sage.

Locker, D., and J. Kaufert. 1988. The Breath of Life: Medical Technology and the Careers of People with Post-respiratory Poliomyelitis. *Sociology of Health and Illness* 10 (1): 23–40.

Lyons, R., et al. 1995. *Relationships in Chronic Illness and Disability*. Thousand Oaks: Sage.

Maynard, D. 1992. On Clinicians Co-implicating Recipients' Perspective in the Delivery of Diagnostic News. In *Talk at Work: Interaction in Institutional Settings*, ed. P. Drew and J. Heritage, 331–358. Cambridge: Cambridge University Press.

Millar, R. 2000. *Researching Life Stories and Family Histories*. London: Sage.

Monks, J. 1995. Life Stories and Sickness Experience. *Culture, Medicine and Psychiatry* 19: 453–478.

Murphy, R. 1987. *The Body Silent*. New York: Norton.

Nijhof, G. 1995. Parkinson's Disease as a Problem of Shame in Public Appearance. *Sociology of Health & Illness* 17 (2): 193–205.

Nijhof, G. 1996a. Uncertainty and Lack of Trust with Parkinson's Disease. *European Journal of Public Health* 6 (1): 58–63.

Nijhof, G. 1996b. Ambiguity in the Interpretation of Controllability of Epileptic Seizures. *Social Sciences in Health* 2 (2): 121–131.

Nijhof, G. 1998a. Heterogeneity in the Interpretation of Epilepsy. *Qualitative Health Research* 8 (1): 95–105.

Nijhof, G. 1998b. Naming as Naturalization in the Medical Encounter. *Journal of Pragmatics* 30: 735–753.

Nijhof, G. 2004. *Ongewoon Ziekenleven. Afscheidscollege* [Unusual Sick Life. Valedictory Lecture]. Amsterdam: Het Spinhuis.

Parsons, T. 1952. *The Social System*. London: Tavistock.

Robillard, A. 1999. *Meaning of Disability: The Lived Experience of Paralysis.* Philadelphia: Temple University Press.

Robinson, I. 1988. *Multiple Sclerosis.* London: Tavistock.

Rosenwald, G., and R. Ochberg (eds.). 1992. *Storied Lives.* New Haven: Yale University Press.

Scheff, T. 1984. *Being Mentally Ill: A Sociological Theory.* Chicago: Aldine.

Schutz, A. 1962. *Collected Papers I: The Problem of Social Reality.* The Hague: Nijhoff.

Scott, J. 1990. *A Matter of Record.* London: Polity Press.

Silverman, D. 1987. *Communication and Medical Practice: Social Relations in the Clinic.* London: Sage.

Silverman, D. 1998. *Harvey Sacks: Social Science and Conversational Analysis.* Cambridge: Polity Press.

Smith, S., and J. Watson. 2001. *Reading Autobiography.* Minneapolis: University of Minnesota Press.

Sudnow, D. 1967. *Passing On: The Social Organization of Dying.* Englewood Cliffs: Prentice Hall.

Taylor, K. 1988. Telling Bad News: Physicians and the Disclosure of Undesirable Information. *Sociology of Health and Illness* 10 (2): 109–132.

Ten Have, P. 1995. Disposal Negotiations in General Practice Consultations. In *The Discourse of Negotiation*, ed. A. Firth, 319–344. Oxford: Pergamon.

The, A.-M. 2002. *Palliative Care and Communication: Experiences in the Clinic.* Buckingham: Open University Press.

Tijmstra, T. 1987. Het imperatieve karakter van medische technologie en de betekenis van de geanticipeerde beslissingsspijt [The Imperative Character of Medical Technology and the Meaning of Anticipated Decision Regret]. *Nederlands Tijdschrift voor Geneeskunde* 131: 1128–1131.

Von Faber, M., and S. Van der Geest. 2010. Losing and Gaining: About Growing Old 'Successfully' in the Netherlands. In *Contesting Aging and Loss*, ed. J.E. Graham and P.H. Stephenson, 27–45. North York: University of Toronto Press.

Zola, I. 1982. *Missing Pieces: A Chronicle of Living with a Disability.* Philadelphia: Temple University Press.

Index

A
Alexander, L., 22
Anderson, L., 99
anticipated, 25, 69, 77
arrangements, 7, 48, 58
attitude, 114

B
backstage, 75, 87, 97, 109
bad news, 9, 11
Berg, M., 82
biographical work, 7, 68
borders, 58, 66, 75, 76–79, 82, 84, 87
Bury, M., 76

C
Calnan, M., 76
cancer, 10, 27, 55, 57, 73, 83, 88–90
Caplan, G., 20
care, 2–5, 9, 15, 21, 28, 33, 34, 36, 41, 48, 50, 54–59, 61–63, 66, 68, 70, 71, 74, 76, 81–84, 87, 91, 106, 108, 114
caste society, 82
control, 5, 14, 21, 22, 24, 25, 52, 57, 72, 90, 93, 106
Corbin, J., 36, 48, 58, 63
crisis, 11, 26, 27, 31, 38
Czarniawska, B., 99

D
death, 13, 25–27, 30, 31, 41, 45, 83, 90, 93, 95, 97, 116
decision regret, 69
dependency, 5, 12, 15, 22, 34, 37–40, 39, 40, 44, 59, 103
De Swaan, A., 37, 88
deviation, 12, 75
disability(ies), 51, 53, 94
disruption, 76, 108
domination, 22, 36, 38

E
Elias, N., 95
ethnomethodologist, 14, 20
everyday, 1–4, 11, 14, 16, 20, 26, 37, 49, 57, 59, 62, 63, 66, 72, 74, 84, 91, 94, 97, 103, 105, 106

G. Nijhof, *Sickness Work*,
https://doi.org/10.1007/978-981-13-0326-5

everyday innocence, 13, 14
everyday work, 7, 58
explore borders, 78

F
family, 4, 35, 55, 57, 61, 94
fatigue, 16–19, 29
Fox, R., 82
Frank, A., 6
French, S., xv
friends, 5, 35, 37, 39, 40, 48, 78, 83, 94
frontstage, 87

G
Garfinkel, H., 20
gesture, 9–11, 109
Glaser, B., 82
Goffman, E., 73, 75, 87
gravity, 81, 82, 84, 86

H
habituation, 49, 72, 73, 75, 113
Heritage, J., 20
homecare, 4, 5, 57, 58, 62
hope, 23, 60, 83, 88, 89, 95, 96, 109

I
illness management, 58
incantation, 21–31
innocence, 11–15, 60
insecurity, 26, 28
intensive care unit (ICU), 22, 23
interrupted innocence, 14
isolation, 12, 34, 36, 38, 61, 95

J
Josselson, R., 99

K
Kaufert, J., 21

L
language, 9–12, 58, 91, 95, 96
Lefton, M., 6
legitimation, 6, 7, 68, 79, 93, 106–109
levity, 81, 82, 84, 86
Lieblich, A., 99
life stories, 36, 41, 78, 91, 115
Locker, D., 21
Lyons, R., 12

M
machine, 22–25, 85
management, illness, 58
managerial work, 59
Maynard, D., 20
medicalization, 62
medical sociologist(s), 1–3, 9, 11, 12, 30, 35, 36, 38, 54, 58, 63, 67, 69, 72, 75, 90
medical sociology, 2, 40, 50, 58, 63, 68, 73, 86, 95, 101, 105
Millar, R., 99
Monks, J., 99
Murphy, R., 6, 94

N
natural attitude, 114
naturalization, 20, 114
naturalness, 20, 78, 114
network, 12, 34, 37, 55, 77, 90

night, 3, 4, 14, 17, 56, 63–66, 70, 84, 85, 89
Nijhof, G., 17, 76, 78, 85
normal, 11–13, 17–19, 26, 31, 34, 40, 45, 48, 49, 53, 57, 58, 63, 73–76, 78, 79, 92, 93, 102, 107, 108, 114–116

O
Ochberg, R., 99
optimism, 88, 90

P
paradox, 5
Parkinson's disease, 36, 78, 102, 104
Parsons, T., 12, 105
participatory observation, 6
partner, 4, 5, 34–36, 41, 58, 73
permanent receptivity, xi
personal sociology, 6
precariousness, 30, 75, 98, 103, 106, 115
private, 52, 82, 84, 87, 97, 111
private life, 87, 103
professional domination, 22
progress, 25, 77, 88, 110
psychology, 48
public, 3, 50, 53, 59, 63, 71, 73, 86, 87, 97

R
receptivity, xi
regime of silence, 97
regret, decision, 69
rehabilitation, vii
Robillard, A., 6
Robinson, I., 76
Rosenwald, G., 99
routine work, 57, 87

S
Scheff, T., 12
Schutz, A., 114
Scott, J., 99
self-occupation, 29
sickness work, 1, 3–5, 7, 36, 63, 66, 72
sick role, 58, 67, 106–108
silence, 30, 89, 91, 95–98, 108, 109
silence of illness, 90, 95, 97
Silverman, D., 22, 98
Smith, S., 99
social death, 82
speech acts, 92
stigma, 102
stoma, 69, 73, 74, 104
Sudnow, D., 82

T
Taylor, K., 9
technology, 21, 24, 59
techno-security, 21
Ten Have, P., 20
The, A.-M., 88
Tijmstra, T., 69
trained incapacity, 2
trajectory work, 48
transformation, xv, 11
trust, 102, 105, 115

U
uncertainty(ies), 13, 39, 68, 75, 78, 79, 98, 101–104, 108
underlife, 87
unlegitimized, 79
unreliability, 101, 102, 104–106, 109

V
Van der Geest, S., 38
Von Faber, M., 38

W
Watson, J., 99
work, 1, 3–7, 12, 13, 16, 17, 23–30, 34, 36, 39, 47, 48, 50, 54, 56–63, 66, 68–71, 75, 77, 79, 81, 82, 84, 85, 87, 89, 94, 103–106, 108, 115

Z
Zola, I., xi, xiv

MIX

Papier | Fördert gute Waldnutzung

FSC® C083411

Kolibri 360 GmbH
Ferdinand-Jühlke-Straße 7
99095 Erfurt, Deutschland
produktsicherheit@kolibri360.de